Hey, Yoga Man!
Yoga Practices for Everyday Life from a Prison Yoga Practice

Shiva Steve Ordog

HeyYogaMan Press, Raleigh, NC USA

ISBN : 0615442005
ISBN-13: 978-0615442006 (HeyYogaMan Press)

Printed in the United States of America.

Dedication

To my teachers, my students, and my friends.

Why I am writing this book

This book grew out of the yoga classes I teach at Wake Correctional Center in Raleigh, North Carolina. Some of this material comes from my blog *Yoga Inside and Out | Insights from a Prison Yoga Practice*, available at:

http://www.shivasteveordog.wordpress.com

The class includes hatha yoga asanas. We also discuss material that covers the breadth of other practices that are part of the 7,000 year old yoga and Tantra tradition that started with Shiva. I wanted to be able to give a nicer handout than a stack of photocopies, so here it is. This book is also suitable for any introductory yoga class, or prison yoga class, or as a support for attention and awareness practice. If you find something here of value, please use it. Don't worry about drinking down the whole thing; just take any little sip you like.

Acknowledgements

Pashupati Steven Landau M.D. E-RYT: thank you for being my yoga instructor and upaguru and originator of the prison yoga program.

Cheri Huber: thank you for being my Zen teacher.

Shuddhatmananda and **Vishvamitra**: thank you for being my acaryas.

Shrii Shrii Ananadamurti: thank you for Ananda Marga.

Wake Correctional Center and Johnston Correctional Institution inmates, staff, and volunteers: thank you for your friendship and participation.

Bela Coble: thank you for early reading of the manuscript and insights.

Lorna Nelson: thank you for editing this book.

Bo and Sita Lozoff: thank you for the books and encouragement.

Justin Mitchener www.perfectionthroughdesign.com: thank you for a beautiful cover design.

Mary Ordog and Johnny Nipper: thank you for the help with the final document production.

Contents

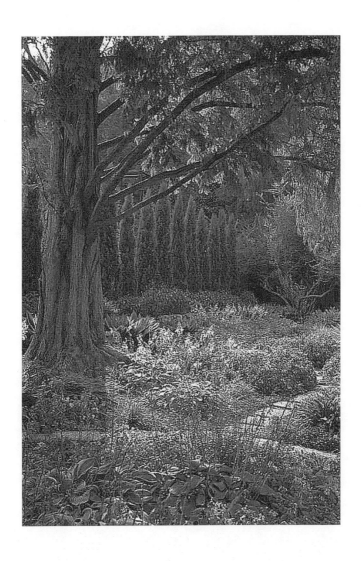

Hey, Yoga Man!

1

This Prison Yoga Program Was Not My Idea!

Pashupati Steven Landau MD, FAAFP, ABHM, E-RYT started the Yoga program at the local prison. He also kept track for a while and found that guys who came to four or more Yoga classes there returned to prison at a lower rate than guys who came to fewer than four classes. The full work and results are discussed in an article in the *International Journal of Yoga Therapy*.[1]

I was a member of Pashupati's yoga teacher training class and volunteered to sponsor an inmate to attend class. This eventually led to my teaching the class at the prison. The experience was very good for my personal yoga practice and for my development as a yoga teacher.

Hey, Yoga Man!

2

Hello world! and Namaskar!

This week has already provided me with some good practice opportunities. I have been teaching yoga on a regular weekly basis at Wake Correctional Center in Raleigh, North Carolina. The class has included anywhere from 2 to 13 people. This week I also taught a class at Johnston Correctional Institution in Smithfield. We had more than 15 people there. Tonight I will be a guest teacher at an Ayurvedic Health class.

Yogic Greeting – Namaskar vs. Namaste

I begin yoga classes by giving my name, Shiva Steve Ordog, and greeting the class with "Namaskar." The Shiva was given to me by an Ananda Marga monk named Shuddhatmananda. In particular, he referred to an aspect of Shiva meaning "he who is benevolent to all" – something to live up to. When saying Namaskar, I hold my palms together in a prayer position and touch the spot between my two eyebrows (the "trikuti" or "third eye") with my thumbs. Then I move my hands down and touch my heart with the thumbs. These two spots correspond to the Ajna Chakra (pronounced Ag-nya) and the Anahata Chakra respectively. The meaning of this greeting

3

is: "The divinity within me salutes the divinity within you with all the divine charms of my mind (touch trikuti here) and all the love and cordiality of my heart (touch heart here)."

This greeting establishes that both parties are due equal respect. It recognizes that a piece of divinity (Parama Purusa, Authentic Nature, God, Kingdom of Heaven, etc.) exists in each person... that each one we meet and greet is "God who has come in this form."

Another common greeting in yoga classes is Namaste. This is certainly a fine way to greet someone or to take your leaving. But the Ananda Marga tradition in which I received my yoga training uses Namaskar to acknowledge the divinity in both parties. To them, Namaste means more simply "I salute you." Namaste would be more appropriate for a sadhaka or practitioner to greet a guru.

I find that there are some interesting effects of this simple way of starting things out when I am in a prison. Starting this way seems to have the effect of establishing an environment of mutual respect. It seems to lessen tensions about talking in the group. It also seems to establish a connection that survives long after the class. I often look up to see a man greeting me with Namaskar and struggle to remember a name because it has been months since I have seen him. Imagine walking into "the yard," as they call the open area where most of the men are during their "free" time, and seeing men lifting weights, standing in line at the canteen to buy candy or soda, men looking around and moving in a way that shows their bravado. Here comes one of these tough-looking people who says

"Namaskar" and makes the prayerful gesture of touching his forehead and heart. The first time it happened, I was very surprised and was brought to full presence of the here and now. I still experience this feeling of presence although the surprise has left me.

Yoga has a certain kind of magic that has worked on these guys. Namaskar is just an outward sign of it.

Pashupati Steve Landau wrote on my blog:

> Well observed, Shiva. They rarely do Namaskar to me except in class. More commonly they shout, "Hey, yoga man!" and ask me questions about the class. I agree about the Namaskar bringing the class to a quiet place, and this works much better than any spoken instruction. It was Subhash Mittal who explained to me the Sanskrit grammar that makes Anandamurtiji's differentiation between Namaskar and Namaste so cogent.
>
> Namah means "I salute," and "te" is the dative or accusative form of "thou," similar to "tu" in French or "ti" in Spanish. So Namaste means "I salute thee," and everybody knows that this intimate form of the second person singular is often reserved for God, or someone most intimate and dear.
>
> Namaskar, on the other hand, comes from the Namah again, plus the "kr," which means "to do," so it means "I am paying my salutations" quite simply,
>
> -Pashupati

5

Hey, Yoga Man!

Sunitha wrote on my blog:

> It is interesting that in India, the two words of greeting are used based on where the two people involved come from. In the Hindi-speaking states (North Indian), the word "Namaste" is popular, whereas in Southern India, the word "Namaskara" is more often used. In Eastern states, they say "Namushkar," which is the same as "Namaskar," just pronounced differently. But both forms of greeting are used for the same purpose – to say hello and show humility and friendship. The analysis of the words by Subhash and Pashupati is perfectly correct from the language/grammar point of view, but in day-to-day greeting in India, I don't think they are used based on the meaning. For example, when I call my folks who live in Uttar Pradesh (UP), I say "Namaste" and when I call my uncles and aunts living in Bangalore, I say "Namaskara." My Hindi-speaking folks say "Namaskar" to me (without the trailing "a"), acknowledging that I am from the South! While greeting Pashupatiji, I get confused, and say whatever comes to my mind at that time ☺ Nice blog, by the way. Having been to the Women's correction facility for assisting the yoga teacher, I know how rewarding it is. Kudos to Pashupatiji, who is instrumental in that initiative.
>
> -Sunitha

Sunitha has some great insight on this, and I heard similar things from another friend who grew up in India. It could certainly be that the method of greeting using Namaskar that is prevalent in Ananda Marga is due to the guru of Ananda Marga being from Bengal. As the members of my prison yoga class come to understand that the greeting recognizes our mutual divinity and equality, interactions based on mutual respect grow. This certainly can be had with Namaskar or Namaste or Gassho or Shalom or Salaam or Aloha. . ..

Hey, Yoga Man!

3

What is yoga?

When you hear the word yoga, you may immediately think of physical postures called asanas that you do as part of hatha yoga. Hatha yoga is indeed great stuff and we do these postures in our classes and personal practices. However, yoga encompasses a larger scope than just asanas. We will discuss the full range of practices included in yoga. But first, let's talk about what the word *yoga* means.

Yoga is a Sanskrit word from the same root word as *yoke*, such as the yoke used on oxen to "unify" them. The word yoga refers to a kind of unified state. Pantanjali defines yoga by saying "Yogas citta vrtti nirodhah," which means "Yoga is the cessation of the disturbances of the mind." These disturbances of the mind or citta vrttis include hatred, greed, and lust, but also include hope and love. There are fifty vrttis. They are attachments. They are the thoughts and feelings that crowd your consciousness and obscure your Authentic Nature. When these thoughts and feelings quiet down and leave some space in between, either through meditation or spontaneously, then the mind becomes like a mirror, and your Authentic Nature is reflected back to you. This is the state of yoga according to Pantanjali, and he explains "then the seer abides in his true nature." Yoga is a state of mind.

9

Also, to Pantanjali, mind means something more pervasive than what is in your head. Nischala Joy Devi translates the same sutra from Pantanjali above as "Yoga is the uniting of the consciousness in the heart. United in the heart, consciousness is steadied, then we abide in our true nature - joy."[2]

Others think of yoga as union with God or union with Supreme consciousness. The word yoga itself means union. Pantanjali refers to this state of quiet mind with no thoughts as yoga. Putting these ideas together, we can conclude that the Divine manifests through the Authentic Nature of each individual.

Based on all this you might conclude that yoga is a religion. Although some see it this way, most view yoga as a set of practices that you do that lead to spiritual development. These practices may be done by people of any religion, and they will support development in your own religion. My classes have included Christians, Muslims, Buddhists, Baha'is, Jains, Jews, and people without religious affiliation. All found something of value in yoga.

So yoga is a state of union. Each yoga practice that you do will have this state of "citta vrtti nirodhah," or Samadhi, as the goal or eventual result. Experience of this state is transformative. Enjoy!

4

Another Sunday at the prison, friendly faces and razor wire

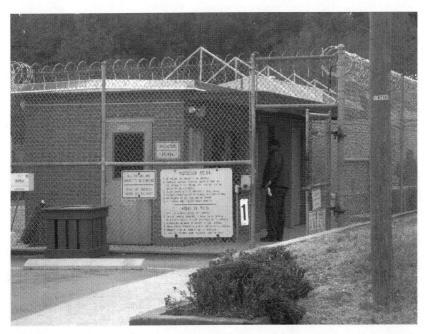

When I arrive at the prison on Sunday, I see this. The gates are numbered, so I follow the protocol. I call out, "On one" – no answer. I can see the window of the guard-house is open, but I cannot see inside. Perhaps the guard has stepped away from the desk or can't hear me or is on the phone or. . .. I wait, centered, without any real thoughts other than, "was I heard?" Then I call out again,

"On one!" This time, a jovial voice comes floating out, "Yoga man!" And the gate clicks open.

I roll my box of gear in, lugging my guitar in the other hand, and set things down. I present my driver's license and passes to the smiling face and say "Hi, I'm here to teach the one o'clock yoga class." But this is just going through the motions. He knows me and what I am here for. He says, "I don't need those," and marks up the book that tracks the comings and goings of prison volunteers. I inquire for the chaplain's keys so that I can unlock our blankets and blocks for class. And with a few kind words and smiles, Gate Two clicks open, and I am on my way.

My path takes me to the back door of the building, where class will be. With my gear at the back door, I round the building to the front. I see the yard, the main guard office, and the men in line at the canteen waiting to buy their sodas and snacks. Lunch has just finished, and I am on track to get my space set up and my people in the building before the yard is closed down for "the count"- a ritual counting of the inmates during which movement is restricted.

I rarely have to do much setup, as the men move tables and chairs and the space is set up quickly for me. I set up our music, Bob Marley to start. Then I gather the blankets and blocks and get things out in accessible places. Then I am off to the main guard office in the yard in order to get my announcement made. The people there know me too, and nod. Within seconds, the announcement is heard from one end of the camp to the other. "Yoga and meditation in the Modular Building," and again, "Yoga and meditation in the Modular Building."

Then I am back to our space. The men gather, and we greet each other with "Namaskar" and "Hi, how are ya?" We talk about various subjects, yoga related, prison related and family related. A member of the class has just "graduated" – been released. Another will graduate in a week and a half. We wait until we have our group assembled and then proceed with warmups. Next some Sun Salutations or Surya Namaskar. Then a variety of asanas. Then balance asanas. Then an inversion. Then self massage and relaxing in savasana or corpse pose. Bob Marley runs out before we get to the balance asanas and we switch to Deva Premal. For savasana I put on a CD of rain with an odd musical accompaniment that one of the guys says includes a didgeridoo, an Australian aboriginal horn.

After that, things can vary but usually include some topic of yoga philosophy, such as yama and niyama, chakras, diet, or guided meditations. These topics form the base of much of what is in this book. This group is often more talkative than I expect and has some very good insights. If there is time we will do some songs and kirtan (chanting). Then a meditation. We end with Namaskar and then put the room back together. I head off to the office to copy my attendance list and turn in copies to the guards and the chaplain. Then I wait for the man I sponsor for yoga teacher training.

When he arrives, we head back to the guard building at the entrance and stand at the other gate and call out, "On two." After paperwork here, we are off to our evening schedule with a usual itinerary of the library, a quick meal, and then a four-hour yoga teacher training class. A quick trip back and check back in at that guard office. A last look at the razor wire as I walk out in the dark to head home.

I am outside.

They are inside.

Yoga Inside and Out.

5

Pantanjali's eight limbs of yoga

Eight Limbs
Samādhi
Dhyana
Dharana
Pratyahara
Pranayama
Āsana
Yama Niyama

Ashtanga Yoga or eight-limbed Yoga is put forward in Pantanjali's Yoga Sutras3, book two. This is the method to fully develop the body-mind.

The first two limbs are Yama and Niyama, which are moral and spiritual guidelines for human development. Yama consists of:

- Ahimsa (non-harming)
- Satya (truthfulness with compassion)
- Asteya (non-stealing)
- Brahmacharya (remaining attached to cosmic consciousness)
- Aparigraha (non-hoarding)

15

Niyama consists of:

- Shaoca (physical and mental cleanliness)
- Santosha (contentment)
- Tapah (undergoing hardship for others)
- Svadhyaya (increasing spiritual understanding)
- Ishvara pranidhana (making cosmic consciousness the goal)

The third limb is Asana, which Pantanjali calls a steady, comfortable posture. Postures have been created to train the body to be able to sit easily for meditation. Usually, when we think of yoga we are thinking of a class of asana practice. These asanas have the effect of lengthening and toning muscles, tendons, and ligaments. They also affect functioning of internal organs and endocrine glands. The endocrine glands include the pancreas, thymus, thyroid, parathyroid, adrenals, testes, ovaries, prostate, pituitary, and pineal glands.

These effects are a physical result of the movements and also a result of tuning the energy system. The energy system is a subtle, intuited control system of the body with major junction points at the chakras. Asanas are designed to affect the chakras and normalize the energy system which then has effects in the physical body, as well as the thoughts and feelings.

By following the first three limbs including proper diet, we prepare for the fourth limb, Pranayama, control of the vital energy. Control of the vital energy is developed by a special process of breathing that helps readjust vital energy in the body and allows the mind to become very calm. Yogis intuit ten different vital energies in the body called vayus. The controlling point for these vayus, again intuited, is an organ in the center of the chest called the Pranendriya. The Pranendriya pulsates in synchronization with respiration. Pranayama with the correct ideation affects the Pranendriya, readjusts the vital energies, and supports spiritual development.

The fifth limb is Pratyahara, withdrawing the mind from attachment to external objects. This is done by a process of retracting the mind to one point.

The sixth limb is Dharana, the concentration of the mind on a specific point. This is done by a focusing process to bring the mind to a specific chakra that is the spiritual and mental nucleus of the person. Once the mind is concentrated on the point, then repetition of the mantra can begin.

The seventh limb is Dhyana, a process of directing the mind in an unbroken flow toward the Supreme Consciousness. This flow continues until the mind is completely absorbed in the Supreme Consciousness.

The eighth limb is Samadhi, the absorption of the mind in the Supreme Consciousness. This is the result of the other practices. People who experience this cannot quite explain what has happened as this state of absorption does not coexist with discursive thought. In other words, the ego is not active when in Samadhi.

The eight limbs have been presented here as a tiered sort of arrangement with successive tiers building upon the ones below. Pranayama is most safe and effective when the body is prepared by asana practice, following Yama and Niyama and correct ideation. The upper four limbs are meditation related, and meditation can be carried out in parallel with the rest of the eight limbs.

Karma Yoga – Watching the gate at Raleigh Little Theatre

Today I am guarding the gate at Raleigh Little Theatre:

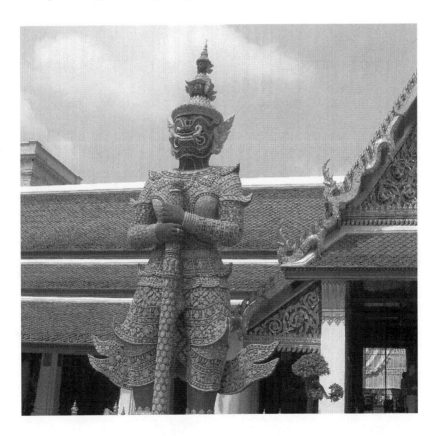

All right, here's what it really looks like:

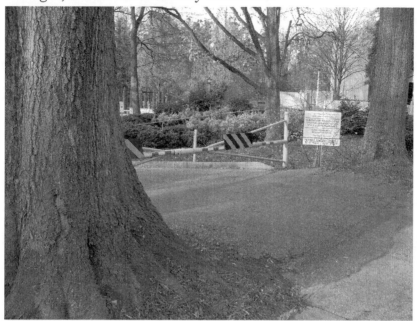

Karma Yoga or Seva (service) involves doing things for others. The things that qualify as Karma Yoga are not very glamorous. Today my job is to get to the theater at 8:00 a.m. in the cold and close the parking lot gates. This keeps the local college students from filling up the lot so that the school buses have somewhere to park when they bring the kids to the morning show of *Jungalbook*. When I got here, there were already three cars in the lot, and now I have the big iron swing gates closed and am manning the gate. I am finishing my green tea from Starbucks. It warms my insides but does nothing for my feet. The sun is hidden by a pine tree. The leaves on the trees are vivid reds, oranges, and yellows, and the English ivy I can see is dark green. I am in the shadow of a 300-year-old oak and another that is at least half that age.

A car goes by and makes for the driveway, and then the driver sees the gate, and moves back into the road and finds a space on the street. I hop up and down. Then I start to dance Lalita Marmika and do kirtan. See the chanting chapter for a "how to."

We do this in yoga classes and at dharmachakra or meditation meeting. Instead of raised hands or prayer hands, I have one hand holding the teacup and the other in my pocket for warmth. I begin chanting Baba Nam Kevalam over and over. I am focusing on the root chakra, visualizing red, and chanting to a tune in a minor key. The movement feels good. I move on through the colors and Chakras. Orange for second chakra and a blues tune. The tea is done, so I make a side trip to the trash to throw away the cup. I probably look like a boxer jumping rope, except I have no rope. A few cars go by. I move on to the third chakra and visualize yellow and start chanting to a sweeter tune, Baba Nam Kevalam. All these colors are in the leaves on the trees. The heart chakra moves my attention to the color of the English ivy, and I continue chanting Baba Nam Kevalam to the tune of "Where Have All the Flowers Gone?" Next is the throat chakra, and I look at the blue sky and so on until I reach the crown and the white of the sunshine and an old gospel hymn.

The drivers have different styles. This guy swerved and made a beeline for a street space after seeing me. Others roll by slowly and pretend not to be looking at me. One guy pulls up and says "I was just going to. . ." but he is wearing an N. C. State ball cap and does not have a back seat full of kids, so I turn him away. There is more traffic now, and they know that someone is guarding their favorite spot. So they adjust.

I make it halfway through the chakras again and am now becoming warm when the first school bus arrives. Hiya kids! Hiya, Hiya! I am feeling good. This no longer qualifies as Karma Yoga. Or maybe it is the fulfillment of it.

7

Yama and Niyama – Guidelines for Living

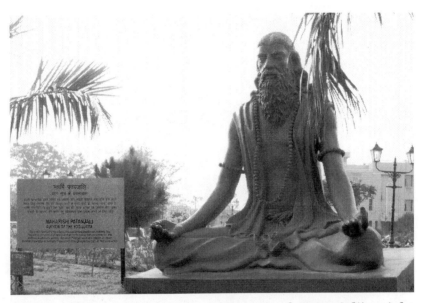

Yama and Niyama are the first two of Patanjali's eight limbs of yoga. Each has five parts. Following these ten guidelines helps build of a firm base for progressing along the yogic path.

In thinking about Yama and Niyama, I am reminded of the Buddhist precepts and the Ten Commandments of Christianity. I believe they were all the results of meditations of fully realized beings.

Ten Commandments:
1. You shall have no other gods before me.
2. You shall not make for yourselves an idol.
3. You shall not misuse the name of the Lord your God.
4. Remember the Sabbath day by keeping it holy.
5. Honor your father and your mother.
6. You shall not murder.
7. You shall not commit adultery.
8. You shall not steal.
9. You shall not give false testimony against your neighbor.
10. You shall not covet.

Buddhist precepts (per Cheri Huber[4] – American Soto Zen teacher)
1. Not to lead a harmful life nor encourage others to do so.
2. Not to take what is not given.
3. Not to commit or participate in unchaste conduct.
4. Not to tell lies nor practice believing the fantasies of authority.
5. Not to use intoxicating drinks or narcotics nor assist others to do so.
6. Not to publish other people's faults.
7. Not to extol oneself and slander others.
8. Not to be avaricious in bestowal of the teachings.
9. Not to be angry.
10. Not to speak ill of this religion or any other.

Yama
1. Ahimsa – not to do harm to others in thought, word and actions.

2. Satya – action of mind and the use of speech in the spirit of welfare (truth with compassion).
3. Asteya – not to take possession of things which belong to others (or to covet things).
4. Brahmacarya – to remain attached to Brahma (the Cosmic Consciousness) by treating all beings and things as an expression of the Cosmic Consciousness.
5. Aparigraha – not to hoard wealth that is superfluous to our actual needs.

Niyama

1. Shaoca – to maintain the cleanliness of one's external world, such as the body, clothing and environment, as well as the internal world of the mind.
2. Santosa – to maintain a state of mental ease e.g. not running to hard after wealth.
3. Tapah – to undergo hardship in the spirit of service; helping others without expecting anything in return.
4. Svadhyaya – studying and achieving a clear understanding of any spiritual subject.
5. Ishvara Pranidhana – to make the Cosmic Consciousness the goal of your life through a process of meditation. Cosmic consciousness involves looking upon oneself as the instrument rather than as the doer.

There is certainly overlap between these concepts. When discussing the subject of meditation with my Zen teacher, I was told that meditation was the key to all understanding. Meditating on the meaning of each of the points of Yama and Niyama and understanding how they are carried out in the lives of enlightened beings will lead to a clear idea of their meaning. Meditating on your own actions and thoughts in comparison to Yama and Niyama will deepen the understanding and move you toward actions and thoughts that are in harmony with Yama and Niyama. One who is living from center, living in Buddha nature, attached to Brahma, living in Cosmic Consciousness, will naturally live in harmony with all these things with no effort and no intellectual knowledge.

Continue attention and awareness practice and use meditation and mindfulness to let no activity of your external or internal life happen unconsciously. Bringing conscious, compassionate awareness to every moment will naturally cause questions about various actions and thoughts. Bringing conscious, compassionate awareness to the Yamas, Niyamas, Commandments, and Precepts will cause you to internalize these results of the meditations of fully realized beings, and cause you to look for these realizations. Having these realizations will automatically point you toward effortless following of these various guidelines.

Vegetarianism can remind you each time you select or prepare food about Ahimsa. Brahmacarya, Santosa, Svadhyaya, and Ishvara Pranidhana can be brought into the forefront of your life through meditation, mindfulness practices, and asanas, as well as by other study and practice opportunities. Satya seems to happen more and more, based on developing compassion through specific meditations, along with bringing mindfulness to your speech. Asteya seems to be a natural result of developing contentment with the present moment and complete acceptance of your current self and life circumstance. Aparigraha is partly the result of the same things that support Asteya. Thoreau's advice is to "simplify, simplify,

simplify."5 Tapah involves seeking and accepting opportunities for doing selfless service. Shaoca involves physical cleanliness but also avoiding things that are harmful to the mind.

This information is just a starting point for understanding and discussion and internalization of these ideas. Yama and Niyama can be extremely powerful in your practice and can bring you serenity in your approach to all that comes your way.

Hey, Yoga Man!

Santosha (contentment) through Yoga – at a Prison?

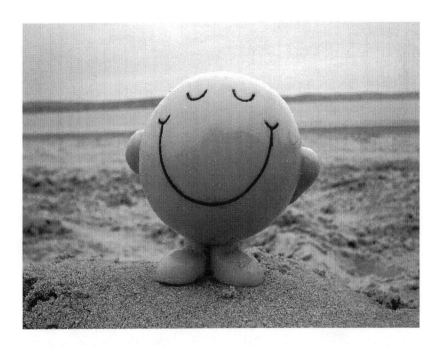

This week at the prison, I talked about Niyama, the other half of the "yogic ten commandments." In particular, I focused on Santosha, or contentment. Santosha is maintaining a state of mental ease. This state involves accepting what you are and what you have, accepting things exactly the way they are now. Zen teacher Cheri Huber is fond of pointing out that "Worry is not preparation."

The obstacles to contentment in the yogic tradition are the Kleshas and the Vrttis. In fact, one description of the state of Yoga is the cessation of the tugging of the Vrttis on the mind. The Vrttis are 50 in number and include things like shame, cruelty, jealousy, hatred or revulsion, and fear. They also include love and hope, which can be attachments. They slip in without thinking and tug at our minds, and then we are functioning in a reactive mode.

Once when the Buddha was asked "What are you?" he replied, "I teach suffering and ending suffering." The state of being without suffering, or dissatisfaction in his terms, is the same as Santosha. When I am discussing this at the prison, I am aware that I could come off sounding like I am telling a bunch of people who have much less than I do to be satisfied with what they have. It may seem that the only way to give this message to people would be to talk up from a more miserable state than your audience. The thing is, this state of "discontentment" is universal. In suggesting that this contentment of Santosha is a possibility, I'm not suggesting that you must continue to live without things or that you cannot move toward goals. What the yogic tradition tells us is that you can move forward in the world from a state of complete contentment and equipoise.

In addition, the idea of telling someone "You should be different" is not my style and not my job. If you internalize the idea that "I should be different," you have simply added one more item of discontent. Work with yoga students, whether inside the prison or out, is intended to offer practices that help people experience Santosha and to cultivate it. The number-one practice for developing contentment is meditation.

Practice: meditation on the breath

Find a quiet place to sit. Sit comfortably and relaxed with your feet flat on the floor. Alternative: sit on the floor, or on a cushion, raising your bottom a few inches above the carpet, or other soft surface, and fold your legs in lotus, half lotus, or Burmese pose.

1. Whether you sit in a chair or on the cushion, straighten your back. Imagine that a string is pulling the crown of your head straight up.
2. Point your gaze down at a 45 degree angle. Let the eyelids hang partially open. The eyes should be seeing but not looking. This is Zen practice style. Yogic meditators often sit with eyes closed. Do what feels right for you.
3. Open your right hand and place it, palm up just below your navel. Rest your left hand, palm up in your right palm. Touch your thumbs together lightly.
4. Now that you're in a meditative posture, focus on your breath. Feel it drawing in and out. Focus either on the point just at the nostrils where the air goes in and out or on your diaphragm which moves up and down with the inflow and outflow of breath. The idea here is not to breathe in a certain way or exaggerate the breath. You just follow your natural breathing.
5. Draw a breath in. Exhale. Count one and wait in anticipation of the next in breath. Draw a breath in. Exhale. Count two, and so on up to ten.
6. As you do this, you will find that thoughts happen. You will find that all of a sudden, you have lost count. At this point, mentally acknowledge that you are thinking. Gently acknowledge this and direct the mind back to

the breath and start counting at one again. It often helps to consider the train of thought as you would a pretty stone that you picked up while walking in a stream. Look it over and acknowledge it. Then gently place it back in the stream and go back to the breath and counting.

7. If you do get to ten, start over at one again. Do this over and over. You are practicing letting go of the thinking process when it starts up.

8. Set a time period for your meditation. Start with five minutes. When you reach the allotted time, gently open your eyes and stretch and come back to the room.

9. Do this meditation twice daily. Over time you can increase to twenty minutes.

Well what is the point here? Here we are considering and letting go of thought, over and over. We are practicing letting go of thought. The idea is that in between the thoughts, we are totally present. In the moment. On the expressway to Right Now. This is practice of being fully present in the now. These brief periods of being present are the state of contentment named Santosha. Over time, more and more of this state will manifest itself away from the meditation cushion, wherever you are – even in prison.

Hey, Yoga Man!

9

Control is an Illusion – Mantra Meditation

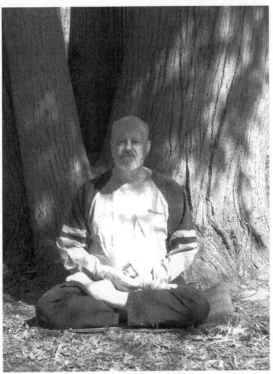

As things go your way, you may develop the illusion that you are "in control." When things don't go your way, this is often a source of suffering because of continual clinging to the illusion of control. Often in yoga, I notice that the various teachings offer development of control of various abilities. This is very attractive to ego because ego is what clings to the illusion of control. I have come to believe that we are reading these words the wrong way though. I believe that the "development of control" of, say, the vrttis (50 strong emotions that pull us out of center) is not so much a building up of the power to suppress or direct these feelings. It is more a quieting of the body-mind that allows a clear picture of the operation of these forces in our body-mind and a subsequent lessening of the development of these states into full blown rages.

This week at the prison, one of my yoga attendees described a situation at his job that causes physical discomfort and back trouble. He has no ability to change the physical arrangement of the work area. He has no ability to change the work process. He is aware that the combination of the physical arrangement and the movements he must make are causing the back trouble. I call this a "practice opportunity." This is a perfect demonstration of our lack of control. It is a gift of sorts, an opportunity to bring awareness to the situation and the experience. Mindfulness and maintaining awareness while experiencing the work time allow varying responses to the situation. Being present while working allows becoming aware of the discomfort during the work time rather than when the backache comes later. Stretch breaks maybe? The key is the awareness. Where does this awareness come from? It spills over from your meditation sessions. What meditation sessions?

Practice: mantra meditation:
What is a mantra? A mantra is a sound, word, or phrase. Traditionally, these have been words of power and spiritual meaning. When you concentrate on a mantra it brings liberation.

Get a mantra from a trained teacher. Mantras are created by spiritual teachers/gurus and energized by them. This sounds mysterious and mystical, but this is the tradition, so if you get to an established acarya or meditation teacher from an established tradition, you can get one of these mantras. It is very likely to work well for you and come with instruction on how to sit, how to visualize and/or ideate to begin the session, and how to repeat the mantra correctly.

Failing that, select a mantra yourself. A traditional choice is to repeat a name of God such as Brahma, Yahweh, Jesus, Allah, or one that is meaningful to you. Remember, yoga is not a religion but a set of practices to support your spiritual development in your own way and religion. Another traditional choice is a phrase such as Baba Nam Kevalam or Gate Gate Paragate Parasamgate Bodhi Svaha.

Find a quiet place to sit. Sit comfortably and relaxed with your feet flat on the floor. Alternative: sit on the floor, or on a cushion, raising your bottom a few inches above the carpet or other soft surface, and fold your legs in lotus, half lotus, or Burmese pose.

1. Whether you sit in a chair or on the cushion, straighten your back. Imagine that a string is pulling the crown of your head straight up.
2. Point your gaze down at a 45 degree angle. Let the eyelids hang partially open. The eyes should be seeing but not looking. This is Zen practice style. Yogic meditators often sit with eyes closed. Do what feels right for you.
3. Open your right hand and place it, palm up just below your navel. Rest your left hand, palm up in your right palm. Touch your thumbs together lightly. Alternatively, rest the hands, palm up, on the knees, and touch the forefinger to the thumb on each hand.
4. Now that you're in a meditative posture, focus on your breath. Feel it drawing in and out. Focus either on the point just at the nostrils where the air goes in and out or on your diaphragm which moves up and down with the inflow and outflow of breath. The idea here is not to breathe in a certain way or exaggerate the breath. You just follow your natural breathing.
5. Do any visualization or other withdrawal process that was given by the teacher.
6. Begin repeating the given mantra silently, either in sync with the breath or not.
7. As you do this, you will find that thoughts happen. You will find that all of a sudden, you have lost track of the mantra. At this point, mentally acknowledge that you

are thinking. Gently acknowledge this and direct the mind back to the breath and begin repetition of the mantra. It often helps to consider the train of thought as you would a pretty stone that you picked up while walking in a stream. Look it over and acknowledge it. Then gently place it back in the stream and go back to the breath and the mantra.

8. Set a time period for your meditation. Start with five minutes. When you reach the allotted time, gently open your eyes and stretch and come back to the room.

9. Do this meditation twice daily. Over time you can increase to twenty minutes.

The point here is just the same as when meditating on the breath. Here we are considering and letting go of thought, over and over. We are practicing letting go of thought. The idea is that in between the thoughts, we are totally present. In the moment. On the expressway to right now. This is practice of being fully present in the now. These brief periods of being present are the state of abiding in the Authentic Nature. Over time more and more of this state will manifest itself in your times away from the meditation cushion wherever you are – even in prison and the situations that cannot be controlled and especially in these situations.

Hey, Yoga Man!

10

I'm a bad meditator – I can't clear my mind

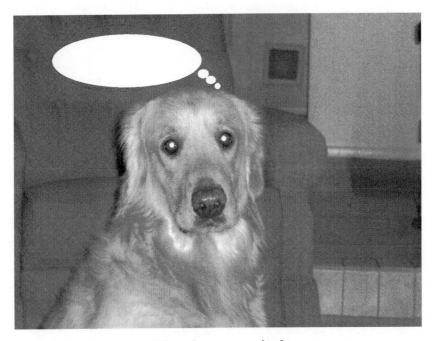

Clearing my mind

We discussed meditation at the prison yesterday. Generally, people teach either meditating on the breath or meditating on a mantra. I have instructions for meditation on the breath in the chapter on Santosha.

During meditation, you focus on the breath, and count. At some point, you become aware that you have lost the count. At this point, the thing to do is notice what thought is occurring, look it over as if it was a pretty stone that you picked up while wading in a stream, and then gently set it down and return to the breath and continue counting.

Over time, you notice that the thoughts will not stop. With persistence, however, the flow of thoughts can slow to the point where there start to be "gaps" in the flow. Chances are the gaps will reveal lower level thoughts or feelings or images or some other form of mental impressions. At some point, things can slow to the point where a real gap opens up between the thoughts and your Authentic Nature shines through. At that point, your mind becomes a mirror, reflecting back the qualities of your Authentic Nature. This state of absorption, experiencing this reflection of the Authentic Nature, is known as Samadhi. This is a very blissful experience.

The recommendation is to meditate for twenty minutes twice a day. You can start with 5 minutes twice a day and work up. People who do this feel more centered and calm during the other parts of the day.

There is another thing that happens. Rather than clearing the mind or staying in the Samadhi state for the entire time, the meditator becomes very familiar with the thoughts that continue to make up the bulk of the content of the mind. These thoughts are not us. They occur in a way that they almost seem to come from outside of us. Many of these thoughts can be from "voices" that don't seem to like us – judging, finding fault. These voices are not us and they are not helpful. The thing for the dedicated meditator to do is to notice everything during this process and begin to "see" how everything is put together. Zen Teacher Cheri Huber points out that there is no certain experience you are supposed to have during meditation. The correct experience is whatever you experience.

As for falling asleep during meditation, this is usually due to posture. If the spine is nice and straight, you can be very alert. It is hard to get the spine straight and keep it straight. Sittting cross legged in Padmasana or lotus pose automatically puts the back in the right shape but can be difficult to do when starting out. Supporting the bottom and knees with pillows or blocks can allow adjusting so the spine is straight. You can also sit with the back against the wall in order to help fight the nodding.

Also understand something. I am not saying that you "should" meditate. I can help people who want to meditate, but I have no mission to go around and recruit people.

Let me know on the blog if you give it a try.

Hey, Yoga Man!

11

They came out of the mist, blessed me, and then were gone

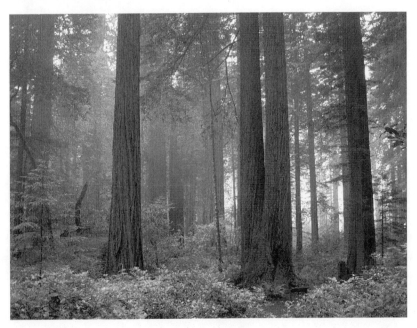

"Raleigh Little Theatre," I answered the phone. "Oh, I thought this was the Rose Garden." "Well it is." Then she asked directions, and I tried to explain how to find the Rose Garden, but she and whoever she was talking to over her shoulder did not seem to know local landmarks like Cameron Village. I finally gave directions from Hillsborough St. and NC State and figured it was done.

I received another phone call from. . . I'll call her Macy. She said that she and her husband. . . I'll call him Olan, had found the Rose Garden and were here but she wondered. . .. She told me of her desire and need to renew her wedding vows with Olan and a secret reason why it was urgent for her. Her secret wasn't awful for anyone but her, but she wanted to keep her confidence and leave others in blissful ignorance. She asked if there was someone available who could be the officiant. I rent the Rose Garden for weddings but do not have pastors on call. I found her desire and secret compelling and without thinking said, "I can do it."

I explained that I was ordained as a minister in the Universal Life Church and based on that could be the officiant of a wedding and sign a wedding certificate. I could also do a renewal of vows and would love to be able to do this for her. She said she would spring it on Olan and call back. She was not at all sure that he would agree.

I hung up and started to sweat. I was wearing jeans and sneakers and had never done a wedding. I am empowered to perform the ceremony, but had never actually done one. Where to get a ceremony, vows, what do they read? Don't those real minister guys carry around some kind of little book or something? I searched the internet and came up with a "Brief Elopement Ceremony." I printed it out. Two pages. The only thing on the second page was, "Congratulations, you may kiss your bride." Brief. Good.

She called back. Olan was willing. She said more about her secret. She started talking about a fee. I said, "No, no, I want to do this for you. . . I won't accept money." I went

They came out of the mist, blessed me, and then were gone

out and wandered around the grounds until I found them walking. They were nice-looking people dressed in casual clothes. I started to feel somewhat disoriented. I talked with them briefly and showed them where weddings are usually held at the Rose Garden. They normally look like this:

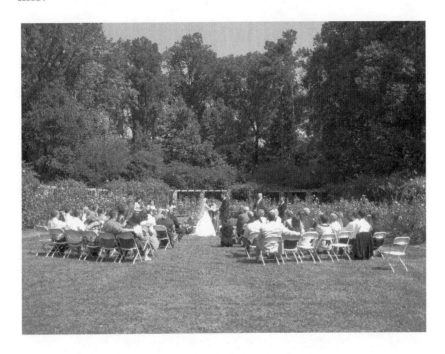

Today things looked more like this:

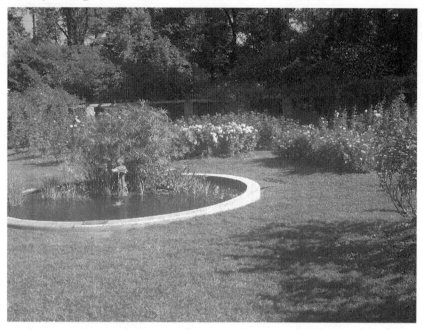

except minus the blooms as it is November, and the gardeners have trimmed back all the rose bushes to keep them healthy.

We stood and I asked names and filled them in on the form. We mutually agreed to dispense with the exchange of rings. They put down jackets and other things and stood together facing the sun in front of the fountain. I stood facing them. I got through the first part about their intentions to wed with their responses very well, voice strong enough. When I started getting into the next part of the vows, her secret came back to me and a great welling of emotion began to crack my voice and cause tears to flow. . . first a few drops from one eye. I focused on my Muladhara (root) chakra and continued on, mentally repeating the bija (seed) mantra and "feeling" the color

red, my breathing got deeper and steadier. My voice
continued to crack as I continued reading, and now both
cheeks were damp. I made it through the reading and
responses, and they kissed. I shook both their hands and
patted Olan on the back and told them both how happy I
was that I was able to do this. I folded my printed copy of
the service double and then double again and put it in my
jacket pocket. I left them there and returned to the office.
Tears were still coming. I washed my face and then sat and
finished up a few things related to Rose Garden rental. I
was watching the clock to be sure and have enough time to
get the box office open in time for our early matinee,
Jungalbook, a sellout today.

The phone rang. It was Macy again. She thanked me for
doing the ceremony and asked if I could give them a copy
of the ceremony. I said I had to open the box office soon
but would have a few minutes and would be glad to give
them the copy we had used. I went up and met them on
the other side of the theater. They both said they had
had a wonderful day and thanked me again. I gave Macy
the papers. Olan shook my hand. Macy gave me a big
hug. By then, they no longer seemed merely human but
had taken on a luminous quality, at least in the right side
of my brain. They asked directions, Olan referring to
Oberton St. which I imagined was Oberlin, and Crabby
which I understood to be Cary. It was otherworldly. It
almost seemed like their existence in this plane was a play
for my benefit, that they only had to think about roads and
directions to continue the show for me. It almost seemed
that the real transaction had taken place when I had been
willing to do them a mitzvah, a kindness, something to
prove that I recognized them as God who has come in this

form. After all, they had found the Rose Garden using directions from me that would have taken them right through the Christmas parade route. They never would have made it through all that traffic.

I left them as they were heading toward the parking lot. They walked off into the mist that they came out of. The Rose Garden is a magical place.

12

Mindfulness – in the Prison and elsewhere. . .

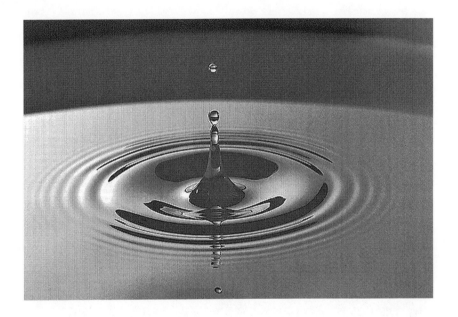

Zen practice happened for me either by chance or by long preparation. I learned to meditate many years ago from the Transcendental Meditation people. Their guru was Maharishi Mahesh Yogi, who was a teacher to the Beatles. I had also read a bunch of books about Zen but sort of had the idea that a person would perhaps have to go to Japan to experience Zen. I didn't know about practice groups or teachers nearer than that. My practice of TM was very sporadic. It offered me tremendous peace and relaxation when I did it, but I did not practice daily or take further training.

One day I found myself at an afternoon session with Zen Teacher Cheri Huber from California. A friend had told me about her, and we had come for some inspiration. It was held in the sanctuary of an historic downtown Raleigh church that houses a Unity congregation now. The church is located on the northeast corner of a park where the homeless gather to be fed by a local mission, and where many cultural events are staged.

I went with no real fixed expectations. Curiosity was driving me. I had a fresh new composition book to take notes and a pillow to sit on. Cheri took us through some exercises and answered questions. She talked on many topics and it was a wonderful experience. The most amazing thing happened that literally "opened my eyes."

All those years meditating with eyes closed had made me think that having eyes closed was part of the deal. I had had experiences of extreme calm and concentration with my eyes open, but they were spontaneous, and I had not had a practice of creating this state. Cheri was talking about mindfulness and establishing a predetermined trigger to remind us during the day to return to the breath, attend the breath, and become present to the moment. To this very spot in space and time.

She had worked us through meditating with eyes open, focusing on the breath, and counting the breath. She had mentioned putting a rubber band on the wrist or a piece of masking tape on a watch band or some other reminder and then using that reminder to in her words, **"STOP and become present."** I had been breathing, focusing on my breath, and counting my breath. As soon as she said the word **"STOP"** though, some sort of shift occurred. All of a sudden the whole world was stopped in the present moment. My eyes were open. I could feel awareness of my surroundings. I was inside the church but could feel awareness that the sun was shining outside. I could feel awareness that the park was outside and could feel awareness of the sounds of the things that were going on in the park. I could feel awareness of insects that were buzzing in the warm weather. I could feel awareness of the people in the park. I could feel awareness of all the people in the church. I could feel **awareness of the whole universe centered in that single moment**. It was a very special moment and then it was gone.

The next morning, I was walking my dog down to the end of the street and thinking about the previous day and the experience. I saw a stop sign at the end of the street, and I thought well, maybe it would be a good trigger for becoming present. I thought, **"What if every time I see a stop sign, I STOP and become present?"** And there I was again. The voice I heard saying **"STOP"** in my mind was Cheri's voice. I was right there in the moment again. I was realizing that this state was available to me at any time, day, or night. It was sort of like having an additional position available on the gear shift in a car. Drive, park, reverse, 1, 2, 3, 4, and now the **"present**

moment" gear. Just kick the shifter into the present moment and enjoy the **"everything's okay"** gear. I started doing this all the time.

Mindfulness Practice 1:

Tie a string around your finger, or put a piece of masking tape on your finger, wrist, sleeve, shirt pocket, or anywhere you think you might see it during the day. Or pick a color and resolve that any time you see it for the next hour you will:

- Focus on your breath. Feel it drawing in and out. Focus either on the point just at the nostrils where the air goes in and out or on your diaphragm that moves up and down with the inflow and outflow of breath.
- Draw a breath in. Exhale. Count one, and wait in anticipation of the next in breath. Draw a breath in. Exhale. Count two, and so on up to ten.
- Keep your attention on the breath and the current moment for a few minutes.

Mindfulness Practice 2:

Pick an external cue like mealtime, brushing teeth, driving in the car, or riding the bus. Resolve that any time today when this happens you will:

- Focus on your breath. Feel it drawing in and out. Focus either on the point just at the nostrils where the air goes in and out or on your diaphragm which moves up and down with the inflow and outflow of breath.
- Draw a breath in. Exhale. Count one, and wait in anticipation of the next in breath. Draw a breath in. Exhale. Count two, and so on up to ten.
- Keep your attention on the breath and the current moment for a few minutes.

Mindfulness Practice 3:

The next time something upsetting or angering is happening: focus on your breath. Feel it drawing in and out. Focus either on the point just at the nostrils where the air goes in and out or on your diaphragm which moves up and down with the inflow and outflow of breath.

- Then name your emotion, out loud or mentally. Say, "I am angry." Or you might say, "I am frustrated."
- Allow yourself to feel where the emotion rests in the body. What feels tight? What feels loose or tired? Are the eyes watering or nose stuffy or running? Do you feel pain?
- Feel it and let it pass through. Let it go.

If the practices seem to be difficult, or if they do nothing for you, put your concerns aside and move on. As your attention and awareness grow, it will be easier to name your feelings and let go.

13

Asana – Building a Personal Practice

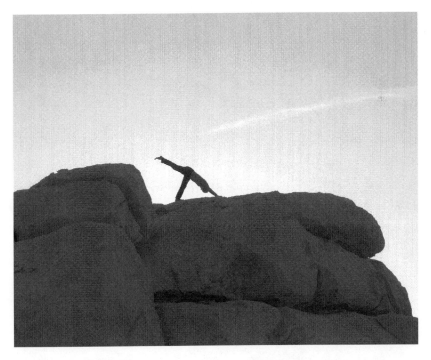

Practicing yoga daily in a personal practice is a great way to develop serenity. To start, think about your day and where it would fit in. Think about constraints – family, work, schedule, etc. Additionally, for those of you in prison, consider constraints of the environment, including rules about where and when these practices can be pursued.

A full individual practice can be as simple as four or five asanas practiced with repetitions, followed by a twenty-minute meditation. Do this twice a day and follow yama and niyama, and you are fully on the yogic path.

How to choose the asanas? Start with two asanas from the beginning of our group class, such as yoga mudra and cobra. Not in my class? Find an asana class that feels good to you. Do eight repetitions of each asana with the breathing as we do in class. Add shoulderstand for three minutes and fish for a minute and a half. Now do the self massage or not – your choice. Then rest in corpse pose for a minute or two. Then sit in meditation for twenty minutes, or if you are just starting, five or ten minutes.

As an alternative, you could use the three sun salutations we start class with as your asana portion and then follow this with the optional self massage and meditation.

It is much easier to start with something very short that you will do every day and then add an asana or two that you want to work on. Don't start with a 90-minute routine that you will do the first two days and then give up.

Make a note card with your routine asana names to help you get through the routine until it is memorized. Use your yoga class and teacher as a resource to get the routine started and fill in any gaps or questions.

Personal Practice Outline

For my personal practice I will start with these asanas:

I will/will not do shoulderstand and fish.

58

I will/will not do the self massage.

I will rest in Corpse pose.

I will sit in meditation for . . . minutes.

Hey, Yoga Man!

14

I've noticed a good portion of the asanas I do at the Prison involve the third chakra...

In conversation with a local yoga teacher, I mentioned that a number of these asanas worked on the third (Manipura) chakra and she asked me, "Why are you working on that one?" I did not have a snappy answer to that. As I thought it over though, I realized that this approach developed from several things and was proven in practice to yield some good results. I have some hunches about why this might be working, so here is the story.

I developed my standard class for the prison with some very basic warm-ups to flex all joints, followed by three sun salutations. Once this is done, I select from a group of asanas that were recommended to people for high blood pressure and weight control. I follow this with balance poses, then an inversion, and close with self massage and corpse pose.

These asanas recommended for high blood pressure and weight control overlap and focus on the Manipura chakra. I think this is because the Manipura chakra is associated with the fire element and within the body fire is associated with digestion. This means that work on this chakra will aid digestion and metabolism. Ayurvedic medicine focuses on digestion and elimination to a great degree in order to help maintain the health. Often people eating institutional food have issues with this area, and these asanas can help balance things within the body.

I have had more than one class participant find the first part of the workout very strenuous. They also report feeling very relaxed after the middle portion of the class. I have also noticed some of the participants shifting in demeanor toward a quiet confidence. Of course, this is a subjective projection, and may be nothing more. But if it is true, why might it be true?

The Vrttis are the human tendencies that are barriers to experiencing yoga or an enlightened state. There are 50 vrttis and here are the ones associated with the Manipura chakra:

- Shyness, shame
- Sadistic tendency, cruelty
- Envy, jealousy
- Lethargy, inertia, staticity
- Melancholy
- Peevishness, irritability
- Craving, thirst for acquisition
- Infatuation
- Hatred, revulsion
- Fear

I've noticed a good portion of the asanas I do at the Prison
involve the third chakra...

On looking at this list I think that reducing these
tendencies to some extent will boost confidence in dealing
with others. I have more to think about here and would
love to have your comments about this on the blog. Also,
you can check out Kristine Kaoverii Weber's post on yoga
psychology which contains some more chakra related
info.[6]

Hey, Yoga Man!

15

Using Mindfulness – Dealing with bad feelings

Okay, you might say, I have been practicing yoga and meditation, but I still have a lot of bad moments. My life still seems to be driven by others. They push my buttons like so many keys on a grand piano. What good is all this stuff if I am still tugged along by every insult and problem that comes my way? You can use your developing attention and awareness to directly examine bad feelings and let them go. Try it. Serenity awaits.

It is good to confront these feelings directly. Often when facing trouble, I have tended to suppress or "stuff" my feelings. They don't go away. They build up in the body and come back later. The body and mind are so integrated by the nervous system and chemical messaging[7] that the mind and attitude are affected by these stuffed feelings. Then in daily situations, you react to this baggage you carry around instead of responding to what is currently happening.

From time to time, you get indications of this karmic conditioning from feedback from others, or perhaps from noticing behavior in yourself that cannot be explained readily from the current situation. Sometimes the connection to the past is obvious, but many times it is hidden. You go through life, then, living a program from the past, not even aware, really, of what is happening right around you.

Breaking free of this programming is very good for health and allows you to experience life directly and live in the moment. Awareness of the present moment is key to feeling good. It is also key to doing things to the best of your ability. Becoming aware of this programming is important to understanding the baggage and dropping it. Some of the baggage may be sensitive material and bringing it up may make you feel BAD. Be sure that you are committed to working with this before you continue. If you think you may examine stuff that brings up feelings difficult to deal with, sign up a support person like a chaplain or counselor to be ready to help you deal with this.

Dealing with bad feelings practice 1:

Get a journal. A cheap composition book will do. Get a pen. Find a quiet place to sit. Sit comfortably and relaxed with your feet flat on the floor.

1. Close your eyes. Take three deep breaths. Think of the worst thing that ever happened to you in childhood. (If that is too extreme, think of something that is just in the mid-range of horrible.) The idea here is to visualize the incident and examine the event emotionally.
2. Take yourself back to the event and try to see it. What did the scene look like? What did the other people involved look like?
3. Can you remember sounds, smells, tastes, or touch sensations? Reconstruct it as much as you can.

4. Now what are you feeling? What age were you? How does it feel to be that age going through this? Where do you feel it in your body? Mine this experience for as many sensory and feeling details as you can.

5. Take a deep breath and name the feelings. Let them go.

6. When you are ready, bring your attention back to the room and the present. Open your eyes.

7. Write up everything you can remember of this experience in your journal.

Dredging up these feelings may leave you with some bad physical sensations. Some physical activity can help this. A walk in the fresh air perhaps. Doing this practice on childhood experiences with the intention of reliving and letting go of negative emotions can be cathartic all by itself. You are letting go of stuffed emotions. Elisabeth Kübler-Ross said that emotions can pass through our bodies in literally seconds if you acknowledge and feel them and allow them to pass through[8]. But, you can spend years or literally a lifetime blocking them.

The practice we did with a childhood experience can be done on other childhood experiences to release blocked emotions. You can also do this practice on experiences in your daily life. Feeling and letting go of the emotions is a big step in healing the upset that you are carrying around. Many people don't even know they are upset because developing a "thick skin" is part of growing up. You don't need to hold it in and have a thick skin though. You can let go and have the freedom to react to the current moment without emotional baggage.

One more practice. The next time something upsetting or angering is happening, do this:

Dealing with bad feelings practice 2:
Focus on your breath. Feel it drawing in and out. Focus either on the point just at the nostrils where the air goes in and out or on your diaphragm which moves up and down with the inflow and outflow of breath.

1. Then name your emotion, out loud or mentally. Say, "I am angry." Or you might say, "I am frustrated."
2. Allow yourself to feel where the emotion rests in the body. What feels tight? What feels loose or tired? Are the eyes watering or nose stuffy or running? Do you feel pain?
3. Feel it and let it pass through. Let it go.

16

Ahimsa. Love your enemies. How come I'm the enemy?

In class we regularly go over the eight limbs of yoga according to Pantanjali's Yoga Sutras. The first two limbs, Yama and Niyama, are ten guidelines for living that might be looked at as similar to the Ten Commandments of Judaism and Christianity or to the Buddhist Precepts. Ahimsa is the first one. It means non-harming. We have discussions over what non-harming means. Generally, it can be taken to mean to live in a way that brings the least amount of harm to other humans, animals, plants and the environment.

In one of our discussions, I had been through the idea of how this applies to diet. The yogic diet is vegetarian with the addition of dairy products. The idea is not to harm animals in order to feed ourselves. We talked about recycling and living with the least amount of harm to our environment.

We also talked about what this means in our interactions with our fellow human beings. In general, the yogic way of life does not prevent us from self-defense or even from serving in the army to protect others. We are, however, asked to minimize harm to others. We discussed this and I pointed out that Jesus asked us to love even our enemies.

One of the guys perked up and asked, "How do you do that?" This is a good question and I feel I owe him a good answer. How many times do people exhort us to be different without giving us a method? We might as well be told to fall upward.

Actually, I have a method to work on this. I got it from the local Tibetan Buddhists when we went through one of the Dalai Lama's books as a group.

Compassion practice 1:
(Thank you, Dalai Lama[9]) Find a quiet place to sit. Get in your chosen meditation posture. Focus on your breath. Count your breath and allow the mind to settle for several minutes. Now work through the following steps:

1. Think of a friend, an enemy, and a neutral person. No enemies? Try thinking of someone who can inspire you to generate some significant level of anger.
2. Examine your feelings toward your friend. Where do you feel this in your body? Allow these feelings to permeate your mood. Now examine your feelings toward the enemy. Where do you feel this in your body? The physical feelings associated with the enemy are much different than the physical feelings associated with the friend. Allow these feelings to permeate your mood but don't stay here too long. Then move on to consider the neutral person. Examine the lack of feelings for this person.
3. Are your good feelings for the friend linked to help or loving acts the friend has offered?
4. Are your feelings for the enemy linked to harm the enemy has done?

Ahimsa. Love your enemies. How come I'm the enemy?

5. Is your lack of feeling for the neutral person because there has been no help, loving acts, or harm from this person?
6. Consider that each of these people has a mother, seeks happiness, wishes to avoid pain, and is similar in this sense. Recognize that had the enemy been born to the family the friend comes from and vice versa, they could very well play the exact opposite roles in your life.
7. Stay with this for a while for the feeling of equality between these people to sink in.

I brought this in and we did it as a group together. One of the men said that the only "enemy" he could think of was himself. Wow! Techniques for this one coming up next.

Hey, Yoga Man!

17

"The only enemy I could think of was myself."
– prison yoga class member

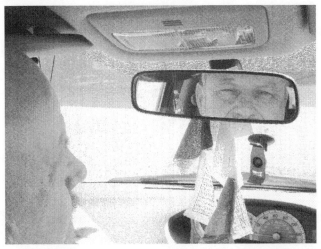

We have met the enemy and he is us!

In the last chapter, a meditation was suggested to help work on removing bad feelings toward our enemies with the ultimate goal of loving our enemies. We are not doing this because we intend to become doormats for the world to walk all over. We are doing this to release bad feelings that we carry around that make us sick. The Buddha said, "Holding on to anger is like grasping a hot coal with the intent of throwing it at someone else; you are the one who gets burned." So the next part of the process is to start letting go of this anger toward yourself and toward others. These exercises are called "practices" because you have to practice them. As you do, you will develop patterns of thought and feeling that make the practice feel more "right." Don't worry if they seem strange or feel awkward at first. Repeat this first one for a while until the ideas feel comfortable. Then move on to the next one. The Dalai Lama's book has quite a number of wonderful meditations to develop the capability of expanding your circle of love and compassion. Consider for a minute whether you are a recipient of your own love and compassion? Are you judgmental and hard on yourself? The point of the next exercise is to expand your circle of love and compassion. The feelings of equanimity, love, and compassion that you develop from this will improve your attitude and serenity.

Compassion practice 2:
Find a quiet place to sit. Get in your chosen meditation posture. Focus on your breath. Count your breath and allow the mind to settle for several minutes. Now work through the following steps:

1. Think of a friend, an enemy, and a neutral person. Now think about yourself.
2. Examine your feelings toward your friend. Where do you feel this in your body? Allow these feelings to permeate your mood. Now examine your feelings toward the enemy. Where do you feel this in your body? The physical feelings associated with the enemy are much different than the physical feelings associated with the friend. Allow these feelings to permeate your mood, but don't stay here too long. Then move on to

74

consider the neutral person. Examine the lack of feelings for this person. Now think about your feelings for yourself. Where do you feel this in your body?

3. Now consider the love of friendship. If you have started to feel the equality and interchangeability of people from the repeating the last meditation, then can you extend your love of friendship to the neutral person? Pretend that your love of friendship is coming off your body in waves like heat waves emanating from a radiator. You are radiating love and compassion usually reserved for a close friend to someone you don't know. Can you feel it? Can you feel this neutral person as worthy?

4. Now radiate love and compassion to yourself. Can you feel it? Does this feel right to you? Can you feel resistance? Look for the resistance. You are just as worthy of love and compassion as a friend is.

5. Now radiate love and compassion to the enemy. Can you feel it? Does this feel right to you? Can you feel resistance? Look for the resistance. Your enemy is just as worthy of love and compassion as a friend is.

6. Stay with this for a while, long enough for the feeling of love and compassion for all people, including yourself and your enemies, to sink in.

Repeat this exercise during quiet meditation times until you feel like a radiator sending out beams of pure love and compassion. As you start to feel the feeling more easily, resolve to bring this new skill into your life during the rest of the day. The technique here is to think about a "trigger" to remind you what to do. The "trigger" I suggest is the thought "I am annoyed." or "That person is annoying." Remember in an earlier chapter the suggestion was made that emotions could quickly pass through your body if you would name them, feel them, and let them go? Well resolve to do that the next time you are annoyed. Here is the exercise written out.

Compassion practice 3:
Whenever you become aware of annoyance or strong negative feeling, focus on your breath. Count your breath and allow the mind to settle for a little bit. Now work through these steps:

1. Mentally acknowledge the annoyance. Say in your mind, "I am annoyed." Feel it in your body. Let it go.
2. Now radiate love and compassion to the "enemy." Can you feel it? Does this feel right to you? Can you feel resistance? Look for the resistance. Your "enemy" is just as worthy of love and compassion as a friend.
3. Now radiate love and compassion to yourself. Can you feel it? Does this feel right to you? Can you feel resistance? Look for the resistance. You are just as worthy of love and compassion as a friend.
4. Now radiate love and compassion to the entire room of people. Can you feel it?
5. Now radiate love and compassion to the entire world of people. Can you feel it?
6. Stay with this for a while, long enough for the feeling love and compassion for all people, including yourself and the person you are annoyed with, to sink in.

If you can just do this a little bit, you will bring more peace and equanimity into your day. You will spend less time ruminating over negative thoughts. You will be able to use more of your energy in a productive manner without as

"The only enemy I could think of was myself." – prison yoga class member

much time spent in gossiping over your annoyances and negative feelings about people and what they have said and done. Even a modest improvement in mood and productivity yields spectacular results. You can improve your mood, relationships, blood pressure, and every personal interaction of your day. This is powerful stuff. When people start to react more positively to you, many good things can happen. Your family and friends will notice the transformation. They may not say anything about it, but they will tell you about the transformation in the way they behave toward you. People will give you things. Your service at restaurants, dry cleaners, and stores will improve. Try it and let me know.

Hey, Yoga Man!

18

Chanting

Chanting is making repetitive sounds. It can be singing or monotone. It can involve repeating one word or phrases. The western tradition has Gregorian chant, hymns, prayers, and responsive readings. In the yoga, we have mantras and kirtan. When we talked about mantra meditation, we mentioned that mantras can be single words or multiple words.

Here are some mantras:

Om - a single word mantra – the primordial sound. Represents three sounds A-U-M, corresponding to creation, preservation, and destruction.
Gate gate paragate parasamgate bodhi svaha – mantra from the heart sutra in Buddhism, meaning: Gone, gone, gone beyond, gone far beyond, enlightenment yay!

Om mani padme hum – hard to get a simple translation of this – compassion is everywhere surrounding us and Avalokiteshvara, the Bodhisattva of Compassion will never desert you is part of the meaning. There are also depths of meaning that would be better left to people like the Dalai Lama to explain.

Baba nam Kevalam – Only the name of the Beloved, Love is all there is.

Bija or seed mantras for the chakras – **lam, vam, ram, yam, ham, sham, Om**
Phrases such as
God is Love,
Hallelujah – praise God,
Amen (sounds a lot like om, huh?) – so be it, truly,
The kingdom of Heaven is within you,
 I am the way and the truth and the life,
Be still and know that I am God
can also be mantras.

Mantras focus the mind and allow ideation on the divine, or some other spiritual aspect of practice. This focus also allows the Authentic Nature to become aware when other thoughts have intruded, and gently come back to focus on the mantra. Thus chanting or singing the mantra is a form of meditation. It is a form of meditation that makes the entire being vibrate with the sound of the mantra. The entire universe is made up of various forms of vibration, and setting up sympathetic vibrations is one of our primordial communication and healing methods.

Kirtan is a form of chanting where a mantra is sung out loud, while doing a movement. The kirtan we do in our yoga class involves singing the mantra Baba Nam Kevalam while doing a movement called Lalita Marmika. Lalita Marmika is so ancient it is said to have been created 7,000 years ago by Parvati, one of Shiva's wives. It can be considered a moving meditation or dance.

Practice Lalita Marmika:
- For the feet, starting with the feet shoulder width apart, bend the left leg at the knee as you swing the right foot toward the left leg, placing the right toe pad on the ground behind the heel of the left foot.
- Swing the right leg back and place the foot back where it started.
- Bend the right leg at the knee as you swing the left foot toward the right leg, placing the left toe pad on the ground behind the heel of the right foot.
- Swing the left leg back and place the foot back where it started.
- Alternate in this way in rhythm with the music (or if you are not in rhythm, just go with it and feel the music and let go of any worries).
- For the arms, start by making the sign of Namaskar by holding the palms together in a prayer position and touching the trikuti (point between the eyebrows) and then the heart. Then spread the hands apart and reach them above your head and hold them spread above your head as you move back and forth with the music chanting. Keep the elbows above the shoulders.
- When your arms get tired, make the sign of Namaskar by bringing the palms together in a prayer position and touching the trikuti (point between the eyebrows) and then the heart. Continue with the hands together at the heart for as long as you like and then when you feel it, you can raise and spread the hands and hold aloft again.

81

Do not worry about being so careful that your toe goes exactly the right place. Focus on the movement and the chanting. Notice that thoughts come as in meditation. As they come, you are free to notice the thoughts and consider them, realizing that thoughts have come, and then gently put them down, and return your focus to the chanted mantra.

One more suggestion. If you find yourself hesitant to make sounds due to the perceived quality or tonal issues with your voice, the sure cure for this is to sing loudly with no concern for the output. Concentrate instead on getting enough air for a resonant sound, feeling the breathing in your belly and the resonance in your heart on up to the crown of your head.

In particular, notice how chanting Om resonantly for a long time in a big voice tends to start resonating below the chin with the O sound and gradually rises in the head so that by the time you get to the mmmmm sound, the top of your head is buzzing. Enjoy these vibrations for their own quality and worry not about what other people think.

Have fun.

Find joy.

Find healing.

19

Visualizing the perfect . . .

Visualization and guided imagery are key training techniques for athletes. The practice is generally to visualize the goal of the perfect performance, feeling the feelings of gratitude and joy about the goal as if the goal were a present reality – to feel the reality of this good experience now.

These feelings improve your life and inform your training. They also inform every action and interaction between now and when the goal is reached. In some sense the goal has already been reached psychically and you can enjoy it from now until it shows up by visualizing it, feeling the feelings, and thinking, "it is already on the way."

This is a way to use your growing attention and awareness to focus the mind on positive goals and situations for you. Replace the . . . with the thing, situation, job, activity or goal you have chosen and rewrite as necessary.

Practice: Guided imagery for focusing on the ideal . . .:

1. Find a comfortable place to sit. Close your eyes and get comfortable. Breathe in deeply and then exhale releasing tension and worry. Do this three times.

2. Now imagine you are walking into the place of your ideal . . .. What does the building look like? Can you see it in your mind? What does this feel like? Where do you feel this in your body?

3. Now you are inside the building and moving toward your . . .. Are you taking the elevator or the stairs? Say hello to people as you pass and allow them to greet you. What does this feel like? Where do you feel this in your body?

4. Now you are sitting at your . . .. Is it clean? Messy? What does this feel like? Where do you feel this in your body?

5. Now walk down the hall to the . . . area. See yourself talking with others. What do they look like? How do they treat each other? What does this feel like? Where do you feel this in your body?

6. Add other steps depending on the situation that you are focusing on for yourself. What does this feel like? Where do you feel this in your body?

7. Now see yourself leaving for the day and the return. Is it a long way? A short commute? What does this feel like? Where do you feel this in your body?

8. Take your time and return your attention to your breath.

9. Take a few moments to feel feelings of love and gratitude for what you have been given. Feel the possession of this . . . as if it is yours now. Feel the

gratitude for this. This gratitude will move from wherever you feel it to all parts of the body to become a memory held in the body influencing all that you are and all that you do.

10. Take three deep, slow breaths in and out and when you are ready, come back to the room and open your eyes.

If you can do this on a regular basis, it will help increase your motivation and improve your positive interactions on the way to your new . . . which you can already feel is waiting for you. Gratitude is a powerful antidote for many problems. This is a process of feeling gratitude now for things which will come in the future.

Hey, Yoga Man!

20

Taking Care of Yourself

What does taking care of yourself mean to you? When someone tells you "take care," what does that mean? Eating a lot of things I like? Lying about watching never-ending reruns of my favorite TV show? Retail therapy, running up the credit cards?

I want you to suspend your beliefs in this area for long enough to consider this from the ground up. Anyone who has actually committed to this program by daily practice, meditating daily (even five minutes a day), radiating compassion, and regular visualizations of the perfect . . . needs to get rewarded. How this happens is the subject of our question. Taking care of yourself. What does this mean?

Think of yourself as a baby. Every need had to be provided by others. Learning was coached. Rewards or punishments came from others. Runners, swimmers, and ball players have coaches. Students have advisors, teachers, and mentors. At this point in your life, you can hire a coach, advisor, or mentor. But what should that person do to reward you?

An answer to this question helps make your practice sustainable and your life happier. Many people have sadness or anger or feelings of lack when thinking back on childhood and adolescence. They feel they were not guided with the love and nurturing they needed. This is almost a universal experience. Looked at from the other side, parents and teachers and others want to do the best but are limited by their awareness, knowledge, and experiences. So this dissatisfaction with how we are parented exists, but blaming the inadequately prepared parents who feel the same hurt and dissatisfaction from their youth gets us nowhere.

As you meditate you come to know a part of yourself that is quiet, watchful, pure awareness. This center, your Authentic Nature, observes thoughts arising but is not the thinker. You may even start to discern that thoughts and feelings arise from different personality aspects. One part of you loves chocolate and wants to eat all the chocolate in the world. One part of you judges the other parts with moral statements, "You're bad. You're weak. It is bad for you to eat a whole mess of chocolate." Meditation shows us how to mentally pick up each thought like a pretty stone found in the stream, look it over, and then let it go.

The different aspects of the personality laid bare in meditation show you answers to these questions though. What does "taking care of yourself" mean? Why wasn't I taken care of like I needed and wanted to be as a child? The answer is this. Your mind's capability to have these different personality aspects allows you to discover a personality aspect of a coach or mentor. This inner coach can parent the rest of you in a loving way and learn to take care of yourself. You may have even done this for others but might not think of doing it for yourself.

When you start to think of things this way it may make it more obvious what taking care of yourself means.

Taking care of yourself practice:[10]
Find a quiet place to sit. Get in your chosen meditation posture. Focus on your breath. Count your breath and allow the mind to settle for several minutes. Now work through the following steps:

1. Visualize yourself in workout clothes with a whistle and a ball cap. See your sneakers.
2. Now see your athlete and think about all the things (fill in your name here) has done. Yes, you are the coach but you are looking at an athlete that is you as well. Look at the athlete as if he/she is another person.
3. List the things that (fill in your name here) has done that are steps toward self awareness. List the things that (fill in your name here) has done on the yoga practice. List anything that has moved him/her closer to a goal, closer to equanimity, or closer to joy.
4. Say congratulations! Great job! Tremendous work! Atta boy! Atta girl!
5. Allow your mind to settle and focus on your breath for a while. When you are ready, come back to the room.

You can do this meditation regularly and that's great! You can also use it to investigate what would be good rewards to give yourself on a daily basis that will help you feel taken care of, rewarded, loved, and generally parented. Examples:

- A pat on the back.
- A few kind words: "Great job."
- A piece of chocolate.

- A visit with a good friend.
- A nap.
- A clean car, area, locker.
- A favorite food.
- A walk on the beach or somewhere different.
- A visit to the park or anywhere different.
- A yoga class or anything physical – endorphins.
- Healthy food.
- Enough rest.
- Clean clothes.
- Get that health problem looked at.
- Time in a quiet spot to write that book chapter (this one) you want to write.
- Time with your child, parent, spouse, friend.
- Read something that feeds your soul.
- Make your own list. . .

Write your list of rewards, coaching affirmations and care actions down on paper. Write 100 of them or more. Pretend you are rewarding another person who is an Olympic athlete. Once you have your list, start to do some every day. There are no restrictions. All the guidance comes from thinking of yourself as coach.

As you do this you can check and say: "Is this for (fill in your name here)'s long term good?" "Does this make (fill in your name here) want to move forward in a good way?" Will this make (fill in your name here) healthier and happier?

If you find yourself writing down, "I love chocolate cake, so I will have a piece of chocolate cake today to celebrate this day," this is probably a fine coaching reward. If you find yourself saying, "I love mocha-choka-frappacino latte drinks at six bucks a pop so I will drink three a day (or three an hour) so I will always feel good until my money is all gone and I am fat and my teeth fall out," then this might not be a coaching statement for you.

The key is there are no rules. There is a practice. Do the meditation. Become the coach. Write the list. Do the things on the list for yourself. **Give yourself at least one reward a day!** Do the coaching statements all the time. Record anything you notice in your journal from time to time. Recognize your great work. You are becoming your own parent. You are becoming the loving, compassionate parent you always wanted. Have fun! Lots of fun and joy!

This fun and joy is infectious. It will spread to the people around you. You will become a coach to others simply by displaying your attitude. You are raising your vibration! You are appreciating yourself. You are reinforcing all your good work. Go Team!

One more thing. Don't turn this into making a list of all the things you haven't done and saying "You need to do these things and get going." If you have only done one thing, then reward yourself for that and keep doing that one thing. Watch what happens.

Hey, Yoga Man!

21

Is the Raleigh Rose Garden an Energy Vortex? - Chakras

Arizona, 2010

In the fall of 2010 we visited Sedona, Arizona and the energy vortexes. What is an energy vortex? Each of your chakras (bodily energy centers) is an energy vortex. In addition, people who are sensitive to energy feel spiraling spiritual energy emanating from certain spots on the earth and have called these spots vortexes. The energy here facilitates prayer, meditation, and spiritual healing. Sedona has a number of these vortexes. Understanding energy within the body is an integral part of yoga. Apparently, many people who know of the vortex claims at Sedona consider these claims "New Age." Some people think yoga is "New Age." Yoga is 7,000 years old and rooted in the Tantric practices of Shiva.

When we got to Sedona, we went to Bell Rock first.

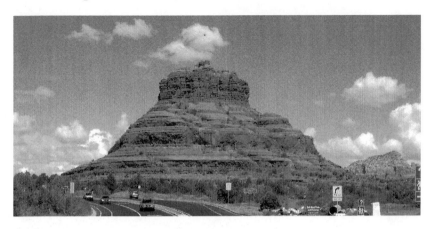

We hiked the trail and scrambled up the rock on the highway side of Bell Rock where the vortex is centered. How were we to experience the vortex energy? There aren't laser beams shooting out of the ground. There are no weird sounds. The trees do look rather twisted. This is from the effects of the energy. We got to a comfortable sitting spot and sat down to meditate. There were interesting things going on in the meditation. A chakra visualization exercise involves visualizing each chakra in turn with a ball of spinning light at each one in turn, using a standard color scheme, and working through the chakras one at a time from the bottom up.

- Muladhara (base of the spine) – red
- Svadisthana (opposite sex organs) – orange
- Manipura (at the navel) – yellow
- Anahata (at the heart) – green
- Vishuddha (at the throat) – sky blue
- Ajna (trikuti or third eye) – indigo
- Sahasrara (crown of head) – violet tinged white

Many times when doing this routine the colors may be indistinct or not seem to come at all. The process may be slow or may require restart. Here at Bell Rock, the chakra colors were bright and true, and the routine developed a rhythm that worked through all the chakras quickly.

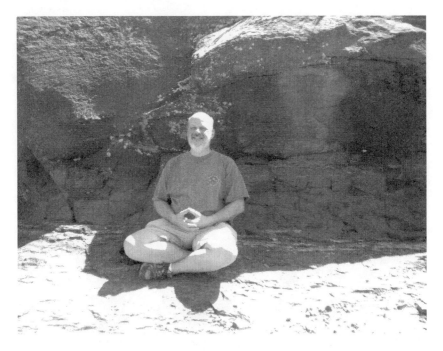

We also visited the Chapel of the Holy Cross which is built on another vortex in Sedona. Meditation here can be done indoors on pews and is more comfortable.

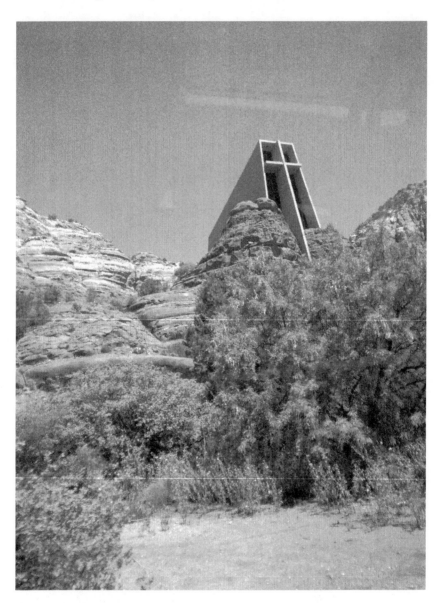

Later we got to the Airport vortex. There is a high rock that was perfect for seeing the whole Sedona skyline. A meditation there proved just as powerful as one at Bell Rock. It seemed like the effects were surging through the body.

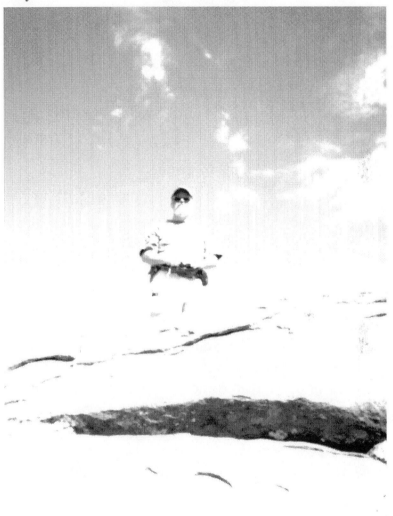

Here was a spot to see a 360 degree view of the entire skyline.

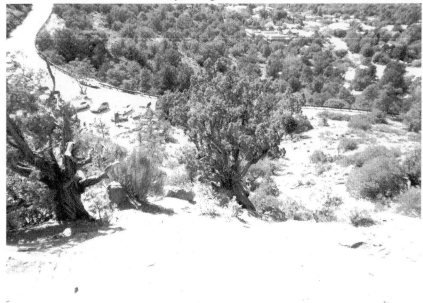

These trees show the effects of the spiritual energy in the form of tremendous twists. There are more vortexes at Sedona, and we hope to get to these in a future trip.

Raleigh, 2008

I attended an event where many of my friends were bringing their various meetup group activities to share with others. A friend of mine there offered to give me a psychic reading. I readily agreed – a new experience. There were a number of phases to this reading, but the one that has to do with this story was this. I was told, "Your energy is not as strong as it should be. You need to be outside more. A good place to go is the Raleigh Rose Garden." Not too long after that I visited the Raleigh Rose Garden for the first time.

Raleigh, 2010

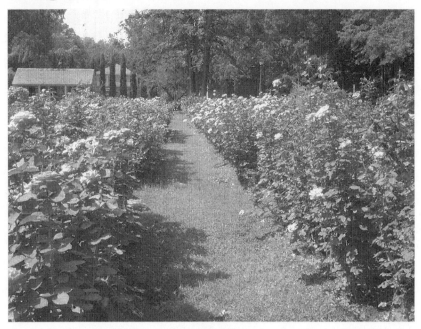

I am now part of the staff at Raleigh Little Theatre and I do the rental for the Raleigh Rose Garden for special events. A coincidence? I have been to the Rose Garden at least once a week for over a year and several days a week most weeks. After returning from Arizona, I remembered my advice from my friend to recharge my energy there, and I also was fresh from my trip to the vortexes of Sedona. I went over to the Rose Garden and started looking at the trees for signs of vortex energy. The oaks are huge!! The cedars are interesting and very large as well. There are some junipers in the garden bordering the back drive facing the office that seem to have the same twists and turns of the trees at the Sedona vortexes.

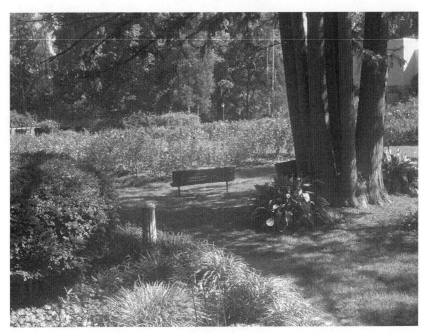

I selected a spot to sit and did the same meditation I did at Sedona and got very similar results. I am not sure that there is an energy vortex here. Can you help me find out by coming to the Rose Garden? I would like people who can feel energy to meditate here, and let me know on the blog. Our chakra chanting workshop there yielded several feelings that the Rose Garden is an energy vortex.

22

Chakra Chanting

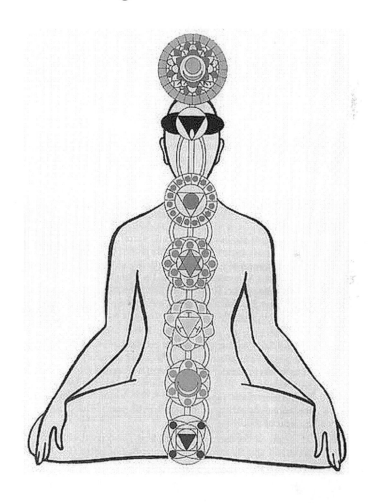

This picture shows the location of the seven chakras. They are, from the bottom:
- Muladhara (red),
- Svadhisthana (orange),
- Manipura (yellow),
- Anahata (smoky green/gray),
- Vishuddha (sky blue),
- Ajna (indigo) ,
- Sahasrara (white tinged with violet/lavender).

These are energy centers along the spine. The practices in this chapter help to build a bridge between the conscious awareness and each of these energy centers. While doing this, the energy in the selected chakra will tend to calm. Calming the energy of the chakra leads to a calming of both physical and psychic processes associated with that chakra.

The concentration points are muladhara (anus), Svadhisthana (base of the sex organs), Manipura (navel), Anahata (heart), Vishuddha (throat), Ajna (trikuti – between the eyebrows), and Sahasrara (crown of the head).

The associated endocrine glands and vrttis are given in the chakra association sheet in the back of the book.

The bija mantras are lam (pronounced lang), vam (pronounced vang), ram (pronounced rang), yam (pronounced yang), ham (pronounced hang), sham (pronounced shang) and OM respectively.

Chakra chanting practice 1:
- After a warmup, sit in a comfortable meditation pose.

- Bring the attention to the focus point for the Muladhara chakra.
- Visualize a ball of red energy at the focus point. Chant the bija mantra lam (pronounced lang) sixteen times in a loud, deep resonant voice.
- Move the attention to the focus point for the Svadhisthana chakra. Visualize a ball of orange energy at the focus point. Chant the bija mantra vam (pronounced vang) sixteen times.
- Move the attention to the focus point for the Manipura chakra. Visualize a ball of yellow energy at the focus point. Chant the bija mantra ram (pronounced rang) sixteen times.
- Move the attention to the focus point for the Anahata chakra. Visualize a ball of green energy at the focus point. Chant the bija mantra yam (pronounced yang) sixteen times.
- Move the attention to the focus point for the Vishuddha chakra. Visualize a ball of sky blue energy at the focus point. Chant the bija mantra ham (pronounced hang) sixteen times.
- Move the attention to the focus point for the Ajna chakra. Visualize a ball of indigo energy at the focus point. Chant the bija mantra vam (pronounced vang) sixteen times.
- Move the attention to the focus point for the Sahasrara chakra. Visualize a ball of white energy tinged with purple or lavender at the focus point. Chant Om for as long as you have breath. Breathe and repeat three times.
- Sit quietly and return attention to the breath for a few moments.

- Open your eyes.

Did you feel sensations in the body as you were chanting? Did you feel feelings or have memories as you were chanting?

Chakra chanting practice 2:
Repeat the entire chakra chanting practice 1, but this time, chant the bija mantras silently. Experiment with repeating them continuously without regard to breathing. Experiment with repeating them slowly only on the outbreath.

Chakra chanting practice 3:
For this practice we will be using the diatonic (major) scale. For those not feeling musical, this is the scale we sing do-re-mi-fa-sol-la-ti-do. We will sing up the scale starting from the root chakra and singing the scale through each chakra.

- After a warmup, sit in a comfortable meditation pose.
- Bring the attention to the focus point for the Muladhara chakra.
- Visualize a ball of red energy at the focus point. Sing the bija mantra lam (pronounced lang) once in a loud, deep resonant voice using the first note (do) of the diatonic (major) scale.
- Move the attention to the focus point for the Svadhisthana chakra. Visualize a ball of orange energy at the focus point. Sing the bija mantra vam (pronounced vang) once in a loud, deep resonant

voice using the second note (re) of the diatonic (major) scale.

- Move the attention to the focus point for the Manipura chakra. Visualize a ball of yellow energy at the focus point. Sing the bija mantra ram (pronounced rang) once in a loud, deep resonant voice using the third note (mi) of the diatonic (major) scale.
- Move the attention to the focus point for the Anahata chakra. Visualize a ball of green energy at the focus point. Sing the bija mantra yam (pronounced yang) once in a loud, deep resonant voice using the fourth note (fa) of the diatonic (major) scale.
- Move the attention to the focus point for the Vishuddha chakra. Visualize a ball of sky blue energy at the focus point. Sing the bija mantra ham (pronounced hang) once in a loud, deep resonant voice using the fifth note (sol) of the diatonic (major) scale.
- Move the attention to the focus point for the Ajna chakra. Visualize a ball of indigo energy at the focus point. Sing the bija mantra vam (pronounced vang) once in a loud, deep resonant voice using the sixth note (la) of the diatonic (major) scale.
- Move the attention to the focus point for the Sahasrara chakra. Visualize a ball of white energy tinged with purple or lavender at the focus point. Sing Om once in a loud, deep resonant voice using the seventh note (ti) of the diatonic (major) scale then moving up to the tonic (do) and then jump down an octave to a deep resonant tonic (do) note.

Breathe and repeat Om at the lower tonic three times.
- Sit quietly and return attention to the breath for a few moments.
- Open your eyes.

Did you feel sensations in the body as you were singing?
Did you feel feelings or have memories as you were singing?

It may not be obvious when reviewing the vrttis for the first chakra that the first chakra is associated with our very existence, and that disturbances here can lead to an intense, unreasoning fear – a fear of annihilation. This can come on when there is real danger, but it can also arrive when there is any major shift in life circumstances. Only Buddhas immediately adjust to new circumstances without a ripple. A person can experience unreasoning fear even from a healing. In this case the person has become so used to having the condition that when it is cleared, the body mind does not feel "correct" without the condition. Here is what to do about it.

Emergency treatment of first chakra issues:
Simply place your open hand or both hands directly over your muladhara (root) chakra. That's right, directly under your butt. Bring your attention to the muladhara chakra and visualize a ball of red light at the base of the spine. Visualize it spinning if you can do it. You can additionally tighten your anal sphincter gently to help bring the attention and focus to this physical location in the body. Take a deep breath and chant the bija mantra lam (lang) for the muladhara chakra sixteen times breathing as

necessary. Listen to and feel how this resonates in the body. Bring your attention to your breath and notice if there has been any shift in feelings. Feel free to repeat this. Breathe deeply and slowly as you do this.

Chakra chanting practice 4 – with music:
In the chapter on mantra, we introduced a sung mantra "Baba Nam Kevalam." This can be sung to any tune. Sung mantra is extremely powerful. It is even more powerful in groups. Think of any sports game and the crowd chanting "Here we go Tigers, here we go," and then slamming the seats twice, and then repeating. The vibrations from this can rock the whole stadium. Bring to mind a crowd singing a chorus of some rock song over and over like the chorus at the end of the Beatles "Hey Jude." It is hypnotic and powerful. This practice involves singing Baba Nam Kevalam to a tune for each chakra. Do this with a group. The group energy focused on each chakra can be so powerful that the clearing of the chakra will allow kundalini energy to rise up the spine.

- After a warmup, sit in a comfortable meditation pose.
- Bring the attention to the focus point for the Muladhara chakra.
- Visualize a ball of red energy at the focus point. Sing Baba Nam Kevalam to a tune of your choosing for several minutes.
- Move the attention to the focus point for the Svadhisthana chakra. Visualize a ball of orange energy at the focus point. Sing Baba Nam Kevalam to a tune of your choosing for several minutes.
- Move the attention to the focus point for the Manipura chakra. Visualize a ball of yellow energy at the focus point. Sing Baba Nam Kevalam to a tune of your choosing for several minutes.

- Move the attention to the focus point for the Anahata chakra. Visualize a ball of green energy at the focus point. Sing Baba Nam Kevalam to a tune of your choosing for several minutes.
- Move the attention to the focus point for the Vishuddha chakra. Visualize a ball of sky blue energy at the focus point. Sing Baba Nam Kevalam to a tune of your choosing for several minutes.
- Move the attention to the focus point for the Ajna chakra. Visualize a ball of indigo energy at the focus point. Sing Baba Nam Kevalam to a tune of your choosing for several minutes.
- Move the attention to the focus point for the Sahasrara chakra. Visualize a ball of white energy tinged with purple or lavender at the focus point. Sing Baba Nam Kevalam to a tune of your choosing for several minutes.
- Sit quietly and return attention to the breath for a few moments.
- Open your eyes.

Did you feel sensations in the body as you were singing?
Did you feel feelings or have memories as you were singing?

The chakra chanting practices offered here are great if done with groups. Find a group to do yoga with and practice these chants with them. The practice of silently repeating the bija mantras as you move your attention through each chakra is a wonderful addition to your personal practice and can be done as part of your daily routine.

Glossary

Acarya (acharya) – meditation teacher

Ahimsa – non-harming

Ajna (ag-nya) chakra – energy center positioned at the eyebrow region and associated with the pituitary gland

Anahata chakra – energy center physically positioned at the heart region and associated with the thymus gland

Ananda - bliss

Ananda Marga - "The Path of Bliss," a socio-spiritual movement founded in 1955 by Prabhat Ranjan Sarkar.

Aparigraha - non-hoarding

Asana – position held comfortably, a yoga posture

Ashtanga yoga – eight limbed yoga, according to Pantanjali The eight limbs are: moral restraint or Yama, discipline or Niyama, posture or Asana, breath control or Pranayama, sense withdrawal or Pratyahara, concentration or Dharana, meditation or Dhyana, and ecstasy or Samadhi.

Asteya - non-stealing

Attention and awareness practice – meditation and mindfulness practice and other spiritual practices

Authentic Nature - the fundamental unity beneath all existence; the ground of being, the witnessing awareness

Baba - Father or most beloved. To His followers, Shrii Shrii Anandamurti is known as Baba.

Baba Nam Kevalam – a mantra which means "Only the name of the Beloved," or "Love is all there is"

Brahma - the one Divine essence and source from which all created things emanate or with which they are identified and to which they return; the Absolute, the Eternal (not generally an object of worship, but rather of meditation and knowledge). The Infinite form of the universe.

Brahmacharya - remaining attached to cosmic consciousness

Burmese Pose - Sit cross-legged. Now move the legs so that they are parallel to each other with the right foot in front of the left leg and the left foot behind the right leg. A pillow to raise the bottom will help to keep the back straight.

Chakra – energy center, wheel

Citta (chitta) – mind
Cosmic consciousness - state of eternal bliss
Dada – brother, monk
Dharana - concentration or holding the mind to one thought
Dharma - one's true nature
Dharmacakra - 'circle of spirituality', when kiirtan and meditation are practiced collectively
Dhyana – directing the flow of the mind to the divine (meditation)
Didi – sister, nun
Gassho – a mudra (hand posture) used in Zen formed by placing the palms and fingers of the hands together in a prayer like position in front of the mouth - with the fingertips at a point just short of the bottom of the nose and then accompanied by a bow
Guru – dispeller of darkness, teacher
Guru puja - an ancient Sanskrit song to end meditation, offering all aspects of one's mind to Cosmic Consciousness.
Half Lotus Pose (Ardha Padmasana) - Sit cross-legged. Clasp one of your feet and bring it on top of the opposite thigh.
Hatha yoga - uses physical poses or asanas, breathing techniques or pranayama, and meditation to achieve better health, as well as spirituality
Ideation – holding an idea or image firmly in the mind
Ishvara pranidhana - making cosmic consciousness the goal
-ji – a suffix added to a name as an honorific
Karma yoga – to act or work maintaining spiritual ideation
Kirtan - singing of a mantra to a melody. In Ananda Marga, this refers to the singing of Baba Nam Kevalam.
Klesha – affliction, there are five: ignorance, ego, attraction, aversion, and fear of death
Lalita marmika – a yogic dance
Lotus Pose (Padmasana) - Sit cross-legged. Hold your right foot with both hands and bring it on top of your left thigh. Hold your left foot with both hands and bring it on top of your right thigh.
Manipura chakra – energy center positioned at the navel and associated with the adrenal glands

Mantra - a sound or group of sounds with a particular meaning which, when meditated upon, help to focus the mind

Meditation – specific practices, attention, and awareness that develop one spiritually

Mindfulness – being completely present to the moment

Muladhara chakra – energy center located at the base of the spine and associated with the prostate gland

Namaskara, Namaskar, Namaste - salutations

Nirodhah - cessation

Niyama – five observances relating to inner discipline and responsibility

Parama Purusa - Cosmic Consciousness; the witnessing, all-pervasive Entity and source of all creation.

Patañjali - (2nd c. BCE) doctor, philologist, and compiler of the Yoga Sūtras

Prakrti - the cosmic force responsible for the creation of the world

Prana - vital energy

Pranayama – control of the vital energy gained by controlling the breath

Pranendriya – an intuited energy organ located in the center of the chest - pulsates in synchronization with the process of respiration

Pratyahara - withdrawal of senses from the outside world

Sadhaka – spiritual practitioner

Sadhana – spiritual practice

Sahasrara chakra – energy center located at the crown of the head and associated with the pineal gland

Samadhi - absorption of the unit mind into the cosmic mind. Oneness with the goal. Suspension of mind. A state of abiding in one's Authentic Nature.

Sam'gacchadhvam' - an ancient Sanskrit song to begin collective meditation. The spirit of moving together.

Samskara – a stored mental impression

Sannyasii – a renunciant, monk, nun

Sanskrit - an ancient language, developed in India. Through this language many spiritual ideas are expressed. It is also used for mantras and other spiritual incantations. The deep, inner sounds of the human body and of human nature are expressed through this language. It is the root of many contemporary Asian languages as well as European ones.

Santosha - contentment

Satya - truthfulness with compassion

Savasana (shavasana) – corpse pose, lying on the back

Seva – selfless service

Shaoca (shaocha) - physical and mental cleanliness

Shiva - also known as Sadashiva. The first person to systemise Tantra Yoga 7,000 years ago.

Shrii Shrii Anandamurti (P. R. Sarkar)– (May 11, 1921 – October 21, 1990), founder of Ananda Marga (*the Path of Bliss*). Sarkar was affectionately referred to as **Baba** (meaning "the dear one") by his disciples.

Svadhisthana chakra – energy center located at the base of the sex organs

Svadhyaya - increasing spiritual understanding

Tantra Yoga - "Liberation from crudeness." A spiritual tradition, first systematised by Shiva. Meditation and other physico-psychic-spiritual practices are integral to Tantra.

Tantric - relating to the spiritual tradition of Tantra

Tapah - undergoing hardship for others

Trikuti - the point above the nose between the two eyebrows; one of the points of concentration

Unit consciousness - the witnessing counterpart or entity beyond mental suspension

Vayu - vital energy - or "wind." There are ten vayus in the human body which are responsible for respiration, circulation of the blood excretion of wastes, movement of limbs, and sound

Vishuddha chakra – energy center located at the throat and associated with the thyroid gland

Vrtti – mental tendencies, vrttis pull us out of center, there are fifty vrttis, see chakra associations

Yama – five observances whose aim is to harmonize our interactions with the outer world and with ourselves

Yoga – unification, state of unity, state of abiding in the Authentic Nature

Yogi - one who practices yoga

Yogic - relating to the spiritual practices of Yoga

Hey, Yoga Man!

Sanskrit Chants

Baba nam Kevalam - Love is all there is.   Only the name of the beloved.

Sam'gacchadvam' Sam'vadadhvam'	We all move together, We all sing together
Sam'vo manam' si janatam	We all come to know our minds together
Deva' bha'gam' yatha'pu'rve	Like the sages of the past at the festivals
Sam'ja 'nana' upa'sate	We share the fruits of the Universe together
Sam'anii va'kuti	Unite our intentions
Sama'na hridaya ' nivaha	Let our hearts be inseparable
Sama 'namastu vo mano'	As in joining our minds together
Yatha vaha susaha'sati	We become one.

Nityam' shudham' nira'bhasam'	Eternal, pure, without blemish
Nira'karam' niranjanam	Without form, without color
Nityabodham' cidanandam'	Eternally conscious, of blissful mind
Gurur Brahma nama'myaham	To the Cosmic Preceptor, salutations

Akhanda mandala' karam'	The infinite Circle
Vyaptam' yena chara'charam	Both moving and unmoving
Tatpadam' darshitam' yena	Which gives me the vision of Reality
Tasmae Shri Gurave Namah.	To that revered Preceptor, salutations

Ajina'na timira'ndhasya	In darkest ignorance
Jinana'injana' shalakaya'	Not even knowing I was ignorant
Chaks'urun militam' yena	You applied the ointment of knowledge to my eyes
Tasmae Shrii gurave namah	To that revered Preceptor, salutations

Gurur Brahma' Gurur Vishnu	The Preceptor which is the Creator, Maintainer
Gurur Devo Maheshvarah	and benevolent Destroyer of this universe
Gurureva Parama Brahma	The preceptor which is the Supreme Reality
Tasmae Shrii Gurave Namah	To that revered Preceptor, salutations

Tavadravyam' Jagatguroh	You are all wealth, Teacher of the Universe
Tubhya'meva' samarpayet	I give my all to you.

Supreme Command

Those who perform Sadhana twice a day regularly the thought of Parama Purusa will certainly arise in their minds at the time of death; their liberation is a sure guarantee. Therefore every Ananda Margii will have to perform Sadhana twice a day invariably; verily is this the command of the Lord. Without Yama and Niyama, Sadhana is an impossibility. Hence the Lord's command is also to follow Yama and Niyama. Disobedience to this command is nothing but to throw oneself into the tortures of animal life for crores of years. That no one should undergo torments such as these, that everyone might be enabled to enjoy the eternal blessedness under the loving shelter of the Lord, it is the bounden duty of every Ananda Margii to endeavour to bring all to the path of bliss. Verily is this a part and parcel of Sadhana to lead others along the path of righteousness.

-- Shrii Shrii Anandamurti

Chakra Associations

Muladhara – red – lam (lang) – prostate (men), – smell – nose – earth – first note of diatonic scale
Vrttis – longing: spiritual, physical, psycho-spiritual, psychic

Svadhisthana – orange – vam (vang) – testes/ovaries – taste/tongue – water/liquid factor – second note of diatonic scale
Vrttis - Belittlement of others/indifference, Psychic stupor/lack of common sense, Indulgence, Lack of confidence (in oneself or another), Crude expression/cruelty, Thought of complete annihilation (defeatism)

Manipura – yellow – ram (rang) – adrenal/pancreas – sight/eyes – fire/luminous factor – third note of diatonic scale
Vrttis - Shyness/shame, Sadistic tendency/cruelty, Envy/jealousy, Lethargy/inertia/staticity, Melancholy, Peevishness/irritability, Craving/thirst for acquisition, Infatuation, Hatred/revulsion, Fear

Anahata – green – yam (yang) – thymus – touch/skin – air – fourth note of diatonic scale
Vrttis - Hope, Effort, Mine-ness and attachment/love, Discrimination/conscience, Mental numbness due to fear/nervous breakdown, Self-esteem/vanity/arrogance, Anxiety/impersonal worry, Conceit/egotism, Greed/avarice/voracity, Hypocrisy/deception, Repentance, Argumentativeness (to point of wild exaggeration)

Vishuddha – sky blue – ham (hang) - thyroid/parathyroid – sound/ear – ether/space/akasha – fifth note of diatonic scale
Vrttis - 1-7 feelings inspired by the musical scale: 1st note/vibrancy(peacock), 2nd note/relieving(bull, ox), 3rd note/quieting(goat), 4th note/peaceful(deer), 5th note/joyful(cuckoo), 6th note/sweetness(donkey), 7th note/tender longing(elephant), OMN - creation/preservation/destruction, HUM - movement of the divine force(sound of the kundalinii), PHAT - fruition or inspiration/theory into practice (practication), Expression(for mundane welfare), Altruism(for psychic welfare, subtler sphere), Universal welfare(noble actions), Surrender to a higher power(Supreme Entity), Poisonous quality of voice/speech/repulsive expression, Attractive quality of voice/speech/sweet expression

Ajna – indigo – sham (shang) – pituitary – beyond the senses – beyond the elements – sixth note of diatonic scale
Vrttis – mundane knowledge, spiritual knowledge

Sahasrara – white tinged with purple/lavender – om – pineal – beyond the senses – beyond the elements – seventh note of diatonic scale
Vrttis – beyond the vrttis

119

Hey, Yoga Man!

Photo Credits

p. ix Raleigh Rose garden - City of Raleigh Parks and Recreation Department, G. Paul Slovensky

Ch 4 Prison gate – Author

Ch 6 Trees in Mist – © Michael Schweppe / Wikimedia Commons / CC-BY-SA-2.0

Ch 6 Wedding - Kayelily Middleton - kayelily@mindspring.com http://www.aweddingminister.com/raleigh_north_carolina_wedding_minister.htm

Ch 6 Raleigh Rose garden – City of Raleigh Parks and Recreation Department, G. Paul Slovensky

Ch 7 Pantanjali – © Alokprasad / Wikimedia Commons / CC-BY-SA-3.0

Ch 8 Smiley face – Russell Davies

Ch 9 Author in lotus – Bela Coble

Ch 10 Clearing my mind – Shiner the Golden Retriever – Bela Coble

Ch 11 Gate guard – © Saad Akhtar / Wikimedia Commons / CC-BY-SA-2.0 Raleigh Little Theatre gate - Author

Ch 12 Water drop – Richard Hollins Richard@richardhollins.com

Ch 13 Three legged dog asana - © Jarek Tuszynski / Wikimedia Commons / CC-BY-SA-3.0 & GDFL

Ch 17 Rear view mirror – Bela Coble

Ch 21 Bell Rock - © Josep Renalias/ Wikimedia Commons / CC-BY-SA-3.0 Author meditating, Author at Airport vortex – Bela Coble

Chapel of the Holy Cross, Sedona - Author

Twisted junipers at Airport vortex – Author

Raleigh Rose Garden – City of Raleigh Parks and Recreation Department, G. Paul Slovensky

Ch 22 Chakras – photobucket Jessica_9oneone

121

Hey, Yoga Man!

Endnotes

[1] "Low Reincarnation Rate Associated With Ananda Marga Yoga and Meditation," Pashupati Steven Landau, MD, FAAFP, ABHM, E-RYT, Jagat Bandhu John Gross, PhD. *International Journal of Yoga Therapy*, 18(2008), 43-48.

[2] Devi, Nischala Joy. *The Secret Power of Yoga: a Woman's Guide to the Heart and Spirit of the Yoga Sutras.* New York: Three Rivers, 2007.

[3] Satchidananda, Sri. *The Yoga Sutras of Patanjali.* City: Integral Yoga Publications, 1990.

[4] Huber, Cheri and Sara Jenkins. *Good Life.* Lake Junaluska: Present Perfect Books, 1997.

[5] Thoreau, Henry David. *Walden.* www.books.google.com

[6] Weber, Kristine Kaoverii. "Yoga Psychology." *Subtle Yoga.* Web. http://www.subtleyoga.com/yoga-psychology/

[7] Pert, Candace. *Molecules of Emotion.* New York: Simon & Schuster, 1998.

[8] Kübler-Ross, Elisabeth. *On Death and Dying.* New York: Macmillan, 1969.

[9] Lama, His Holiness the Dalai and Jeffrey Hopkins Phd. *How to Expand Love.* New York: Atria, 2005.

[10] Huber, Cheri. *Making a Change for Good.* Boulder: Shambhala, 2007.

8954876R0

Made in the USA
Charleston, SC
29 July 2011